Praise for Gena Lee Nolin from thyroid patients

"Gena Lee, you may have saved many lives on TV, but you're doing it for real! Thyroid Sexy has changed my life and taught me how to live again. Two words: 'My Hero!'"

—*Jamie Kurtz*

"I cannot begin to tell you how inspiring you and your advocacy have been to me. I am finally living the healthy life I've longed for simply because of you."

—*Donna Cates*

"Your truth, honesty, and courage have been so valued. Thank you, Gena, for educating me and helping me to know I am not alone."

—*Kelli Thomas*

"You are amazing and strong! You've taught me to stand up and face this disease head on. I can't thank you enough for being our voice."

—*Jessica Kress*

"Gena, thank you for making me fight! I won and I'm living again!"

—*Marci Teers*

"For years I suffered and didn't have the tools or confidence to talk to my doctor. Gena, you've changed my life through your advocacy. You've given us a voice to stand up to thyroid disease."

—*Barbara Botts*

"Gena, you've literally saved my life! I've been able to help others now because of the information I've got from Thyroid Sexy. Thank you!"

—*Marilyn Foley*

"Thyroid Sexy is a part of my daily routine. You've provided a safe yet very knowledgeable environment for those who suffer. Gena Lee Nolin is a true life saver!"

—*Megan Nicholson*

"What a gift you've given us by telling your story! I can't tell you how much I've learned by your advocacy through your page. Love Thyroid Sexy and Gena Lee!"

—*Jerri Zingg*

"When fighting this disease it takes people like you paving the way for us. I took my letter from Thyroid Sexy that you wrote and my doctor finally listened. Now, that's just genius. So grateful—thank you!"

—*Lacey McKinney*

"Gena, I now have hope, when I never did. I have strength, when I was weak and helpless. Yes, I have a voice because of you! You've changed so many lives because of what you're doing."

—*Jackie Benson*

Praise for Mary Shomon from thyroid patients

"Mary Shomon is our lighthouse—a shining beacon of light through the thyroid fog."

—*Annette I.*

"When I was diagnosed four years ago with hypothyroidism, I was clueless. I was also in no shape, mentally/physically/spiritually, to defend myself or have an inkling of understanding of what was going on with me. Thank you, Mary Shomon, for she has given me so much of my life back, empowered me, understood me like no one else. Her website, books, and Facebook page have literally saved my life."

—*Cindy H.*

"As an integrative functional metabolic medicine specialist, I find Mary Shomon's information, knowledge, compassion, and drive to educate those patients in need, as well as physicians whose heads are in the sand, to be an invaluable Godsend!"

—*Aldino P.*

"Quite frankly, Mary Shomon saved my life. Without Mary's courage to research and post her information, I wouldn't be here. I would have followed a doctor's bad advice and I would have died . . . either by low thyroid or from my own hand at the hopelessness that doctor's recommendations would have left me with."

—*Angela G.*

"I'm a nurse married to a physician, so I can get my hands on lots of medical info, but when I became hypothyroid, it was Mary's book that was the most helpful and informative. I read it cover to cover several times, and rely heavily on the info on her website and Facebook page. When I need to interpret lab results or symptoms, I consult Mary's books . . . before the doctor."

—Lorraine M.

"Mary Shomon gives me hope that one day we will have the medical care we all deserve. She inspires me to stay on top of my health, to stay informed. Thank you, Mary, for so much hard work and never giving up and fighting the fight publically where most of us can't."

—Amy R.

The Thyroid Diet Revolution

The Menopause Thyroid Solution

Living Well with Hypothyroidism

Living Well with Graves' Disease and Hyperthyroidism

The Thyroid Hormone Breakthrough

The Thyroid Diet

The Thyroid Guide to Hair Loss

Living Well with Autoimmune Disease

Living Well with Chronic Fatigue Syndrome and Fibromyalgia

What Your Doctor May Not Tell You About Parkinson's Disease

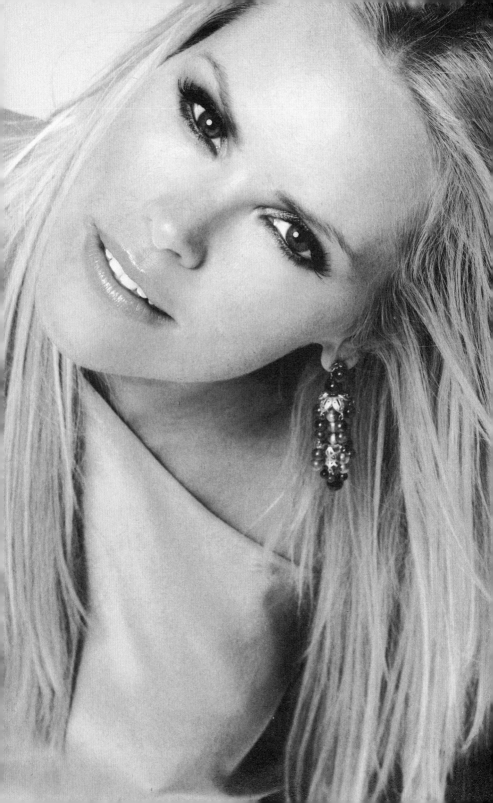

BEAUTIFUL
INSIDE AND OUT

*Conquering Thyroid Disease with
a Healthy, Happy, "Thyroid Sexy" Life*

GENA LEE NOLIN
and MARY SHOMON

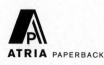

ATRIA PAPERBACK

NEW YORK LONDON TORONTO SYDNEY NEW DELHI

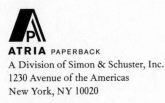

ATRIA PAPERBACK

A Division of Simon & Schuster, Inc.
1230 Avenue of the Americas
New York, NY 10020

First Atria paperback edition October 2013

ATRIA PAPERBACK and colophon are trademarks of Simon & Schuster, Inc.

For information about special discounts for bulk purchases, please contact Simon & Schuster Special Sales at 1-866-506-1949 or business@simonandschuster.com.

The Simon & Schuster Speakers Bureau can bring authors to your live event. For more information or to book an event contact the Simon & Schuster Speakers Bureau at 1-866-248-3049 or visit our website at www.simonspeakers.com.

Photographs on pages vi, 55, 191, and 265 by Phyllis Lane. Photograph on page xxiii courtesy of Mary J. Shomon. Photograph on page 243 by Spencer Fahlman. All other photographs courtesy of Gena Lee Nolin.

Designed by Ruth Lee-Mui

Manufactured in the United States of America

10   9   8   7   6   5   4   3   2   1

Library of Congress Cataloging-in-Publication Data
Nolin, Gena Lee.
   Beautiful inside and out : conquering thyroid disease with a healthy, happy, "thyroid sexy" life / by Gena Lee Nolin and Mary J. Shomon.—First Atria paperback edition.
       p.   cm— (Atria nonfiction original trade)
Includes bibliographical references and index.
   1. Nolin, Gena Lee—Health. 2. Television actors and actresses—United States—Biography. 3. Thyroid gland—Diseases—Popular works. 4. Hypothyroidism—Popular works. 5. Sexual health—Popular works. I. Shomon, Mary J. II. Title.
RC655.N65 2013
616.4'40092—dc23
[B]
                                                            2013009632

ISBN 978-1-4516-8722-4
ISBN 978-1-4516-8723-1 (ebook)

Disclaimer

This publication contains the opinions and ideas of its authors. It is intended to provide helpful and informative material on the subjects addressed in the publication. It is sold with the understanding that the author and publisher are not engaged in rendering medical, health, or any other kind of personal or professional services in the book. The reader should consult his or her medical, health, or other competent professional before adopting any of the suggestions in this book or drawing inferences from it.

The authors and publisher specifically disclaim all responsibility for any liability, loss, or risk, personal or otherwise, which is incurred as a consequence, directly or indirectly, of the use and applications of any of the contents of this book.

I dedicate this book to my loving family.

———

*My ever-supporting husband, Cale,
who loves me unconditionally and
to my beautiful children who continue to
fill my life with sunshine and laughter.*
—GENA LEE NOLIN

———

*Without my faith in God,
this book wouldn't be in your hands.*
—MARY SHOMON

Wheresoever you go, go with all your heart.

—CONFUCIUS

Contents

PART 3

GOING FORWARD

Foreword

Can you imagine having to wear a small red bathing suit on television every week while battling a slow thyroid?

Perhaps you recall seeing Gena Lee Nolin, back when she was rocking her red bathing suit and running with the buoys on *Baywatch*. She appeared to have it all—Hollywood glamour, a handsome husband, and beautiful children.

She looked amazing, but she felt run-down. For years, she worked out twice as much as her colleagues, and still gained weight. Her metabolism—the rate at which one burns calories—seemed to grind to a halt. She was young yet experienced profound brain fog and joint pain. Even her hair turned brittle and then fell out. She was too young to feel so old.

JUST TEST THE WOMAN

Doctors called it depression and put her on antidepressants. They claimed that her abnormal heart rhythm, also thyroid-related, required complicated medications.

This pattern went on for years—decades, actually—before

Gena's thyroid issues were finally diagnosed as Hashimoto's disease, an autoimmune condition that causes your immune system to attack the thyroid.

I don't blame the physicians. They are not ignorant. Rather, they were trained in the same ailing system that I also trained in—one in which we are taught to suspect that women who gain weight have a lack of willpower, not a thyroid problem. And I have been fortunate to receive one of the best medical educations possible.

Fortunately, Gena Lee Nolin and coauthor Mary Shomon have written the defining book about their experiences, and it's my honor to introduce you to them. Mary Shomon is a superstar in her own right—she is the *New York Times* bestselling author of *The Thyroid Diet*. She is the fiercest patient advocate I know, and you can trust her more than you can most doctors as an authority on all things thyroid. She has been helping patients for more than fifteen years in her advocacy and community-building online and in one-on-one coaching.

THYROID PROBLEMS ARE
REACHING EPIDEMIC PROPORTIONS

Gena's story is stunning, but it's also more common than you might think, except for the part about the red bathing suit.

Ironically, the lifeguard needed a lifeguard, or at least a sympathetic and professional ear. Gena needed a physician who would listen carefully to her symptoms and perform the basic detective work that would have saved her years of struggle, desperate dieting, and risky and unnecessary medications, and gotten her back on her feet again with her health.

Thyropause 101

Millions of women experience the weight gain, crushing fatigue, and moodiness of low thyroid function, yet are dismissed by their physicians with a pat on the shoulder—and told in a patronizing tone that they're just getting older, or that life is stressful, or that perhaps they should simply exercise more and eat less, all of which leaves women cold.

Rule of Engagement #1. Do not dismiss a woman with weight gain, fatigue, and mood issues until you check her damn thyroid.

When I was in my twenties and training to be a physician, I thought that thyroid problems mostly struck middle-aged women. Now that I'm middle-aged and a board-certified physician, I recognize that thyroid disease often strikes younger women. Many women like Gena suffer from thyroid imbalance, but both the women themselves and their doctors don't look for it, and it's too easy to blame other problems—you're a busy mom, you've got so much that you're juggling, you travel a lot, and no wonder you're so tired.

Rule of Engagement #2. Consider thyroid testing sooner rather than later, particularly for younger women. Have a high index of suspicion. Assume the worst until proven otherwise.

Gena is the first celebrity to speak out and truly own her thyroid problem, and she's willing to go on record about how she suffered in silence for years while trying to succeed in an industry that is grueling in its emphasis on physical appearance, weight, and external beauty. Gena looked like an amazing celebrity package, yet she was pushing a rock up a hill with her slow metabolism and pleas for help from an unresponsive medical establishment. She is a courageous whistle-blower exposing a failing health care system where women are still blamed for problems that often have a biological basis.

I receive blank stares when I talk about younger women experiencing thyroid problems. People don't want to talk about thyroid disease—perhaps because public perception is that it's associated with middle-aged women, weight gain, fatigue, hair loss, depression, low sex drive—but Gena and Mary are creating a new conversation and openness about the thyroid. Together, they are validating the importance of being a squeaky wheel when it comes to your health, and that it's not only acceptable to go public with your own stories of being dismissed or ignored by conventional medicine, but it just might be your sacred duty. In the process, you might be similarly helping women regain their voice, mojo, positive self-image, energy, happy mood, and sex drive, and last but not least, rock their locks.

Reading this book feels like you're out with your best girlfriends for a glass of wine or mug of hot, soothing tea. We all know the glorious feeling of being with our wiser girlfriends who have been through a challenging experience and are happy to shepherd us through it—to share their knowledge so we don't have to go through it alone. Gena and Mary will tell you honestly about the twists and turns, the shortcuts and the heartaches, the tips about everything from finding a great doctor to dealing with sparse eyebrows, about going gluten free, and the challenging work of rebuilding a lagging sex life.

We all need a lifeguard, and fortunately, Gena Lee Nolin and Mary Shomon have stepped up to lead us. They are a courageous duo, willing to speak out about the life-altering importance of speaking your truth, even when it runs against the prevailing medical opinion.

I stand with them . . . as long as I don't have to wear a red bathing suit!

Sara Gottfried, MD
Berkeley, California

Foreword

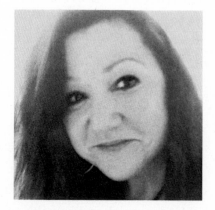

I was one of the lucky ones. Getting a thyroid diagnosis took me only a few months. It was 1994, and I had just gotten engaged. I made a few visits to the doctor, each time with a new complaint: one time it was fatigue, next a new feeling of mild depression, and finally, weight gain. I was eating less and exercising, but the weight was steadily piling on. The weight gain was especially frustrating—every time I went for a dress fitting, they had to let my dress out a size. It was definitely not a situation any future bride wants to experience.

On my third visit to the doctor in several months, she mentioned that she wanted to check out my thyroid. At that point, I really didn't know what the thyroid was, what it did, or even where it was located. I had a vague memory of an aunt who had a goiter, but that was the sum total of my knowledge about thyroid disease.

I remember getting the phone call—a message left on the answering machine. "Your thyroid is low, so I'm calling in a prescription." I was thrilled. Here I had the answer to my health issues, and clearly, once I filled my prescription and started taking my pills, I would quickly return to normal.

I couldn't have been more wrong.

Despite starting on thyroid medication, I continued to struggle with weight gain, fatigue, and moodiness, and new symptoms began to appear. My joints ached, my hair was shedding so much I could stuff pillows with what was lost, and I had mysterious headaches. I was certain that the doctors had missed a serious diagnosis.

I ended up with a series of new tests, more visits to the doctor, even an MRI, and was pronounced fine. But I didn't feel fine.

It was then that I realized how urgent it was that I learn about my thyroid disease, and learn it fast. My health, energy, and quality of life all depended on it.

This was a challenge. It's already easy to forget, but in 1995, few of us had access to the Internet, people didn't regularly "google" their medical conditions, doctors told us what to do and when to do it, and we rarely if ever questioned their authority or capabilities.

I started at the local library, where I found one short book, written probably ten or more years earlier, that talked about thyroid disease and explained how easy it was to diagnose and treat. It was, not surprisingly, written by a middle-aged male doctor.

My next step was the Internet. In those days, you got one of the free AOL disks and signed on to the AOL message boards and the Usenet support groups. Creeping along at glacial speeds—I had time to go get a cup of coffee while even a single page downloaded—I discovered that there were already some groups of fellow thyroid patients who were struggling with the same questions I was facing. Why weren't we feeling well on our treatments? Why did we continue to have symptoms? How could we feel better? What options were out there to try? We were all struggling to find answers to these questions.

I quickly jumped into the discussions and realized that thyroid disease was not the "easy to diagnose, easy to treat" walk in the park that many doctors had been suggesting. There were different medications to try, lifestyle changes, supplements, dietary modifications—and a whole world of fellow patients who were being told that our problems were in our heads, and so we should just take our pills, stop complaining, and, by the way, "quit eating so much!"

I started a simple web page—Frequently Asked Questions about thyroid issues—and began interacting with other patients and helping answer questions from people who were newly diagnosed. As more people got online, it seemed that there was a never-ending stream of people, new to thyroid disease, who were confused, frightened, and looking for answers.

In 1996, I signed up to participate in a new service, called the Mining Company, where I would create from scratch the content for a website dedicated to thyroid disease. In those early Internet days, the editors—who were all healthy young twentysomethings working eighteen-hour days glued to computers and fueled by caffeine—laughed at my topic area. They were willing to give it a try, but they expected the thyroid topic area to fizzle out quickly. Instead, it became one of the company's most-visited topic areas and soon became a key site on the Internet. Along the way, the

Mining Company changed its name to About.com and was bought by the *New York Times*, and my Thyroid.About.com site became one of the top health sites at About, and a leading thyroid site on the Internet.

The success of the site demonstrated something that I knew all along: there was very little information available about thyroid disease from the medical world, and what was out there tended to downplay thyroid symptoms, simplify treatments, and in the end, put the blame on the patients if they didn't feel well after treatment. Thyroid patients were, therefore, desperate for advice, ideas, answers, and information—and they were clearly not getting much of it from their doctors.

Along the way, as I was learning from other patients, my own doctor, research, journal articles, and other practitioners I interviewed, I was discovering new ways to approach thyroid disease, and I was able to map out strategies that worked to slowly resolve my symptoms. I tried different medications, changed my diet, added supplements, and felt better over time.

Each time I learned something new, I shared it through the website and through newsletters I began publishing for patients.

Even though those AOL disks were everywhere, many people were still not online during the late 1990s. At the same time, I felt more strongly than ever that my thyroid advocacy work was becoming a mission—an obligation—and that I had to reach out to other thyroid patients to help them avoid the fear, the turmoil, and the wrong turns along the path to diagnosis and successful treatment. So I wrote my first health book, *Living Well with Hypothyroidism*, and it was published by HarperCollins in 2000. I wanted to make sure that even those who never went near a computer would be able to get the information they needed.

The book sent shock waves into the thyroid world. Patients loved it, many endocrinologists cursed my name, and thyroid disease started to create a media buzz. Doctors and other health writers rushed to start writing about thyroid disease. More articles about thyroid disease started to appear in women's magazines. Meanwhile, I continued building the website, while writing more books, and over the next decade, published the books *The Thyroid Diet Revolution, Living Well with Graves' Disease and Hyperthyroidism, Living Well with Autoimmune Disease, Living Well with Chronic Fatigue Syndrome and Fibromyalgia, The Thyroid Hormone Breakthrough, The Menopause Thyroid Solution*, and my *New York Times* bestseller, *The Thyroid Diet*. I was contacted by magazine writers, radio shows, television news producers, and newspaper reporters to present the patient perspective on thyroid disease, and as my writing role expanded into thyroid patient advocacy, I did hundreds of interviews a year.

Later in the decade, the social media explosion began, and I jumped into Twitter and Facebook, to expand awareness in those areas as well.

On Twitter, I found out that *My Big Fat Greek Wedding* writer and star Nia Vardalos was a thyroid patient and fan of my site. I connected with doctors and other patients and joined an amazing global conversation.

I built a Thyroid Support page on Facebook, now home to more than 20,000 thyroid patients, and an amazing community developed. Patients helped patients and shared experiences, resources, names of practitioners, and above all, the compassion and understanding that were in short supply in the medical world.

And it was on the pages of my Facebook Thyroid Support group that I first "met" Gena Lee Nolin.

With thousands of participants, it's hard to keep track of all the new faces, but Gena stood out from the start. She posted some sharp questions and some supportive comments. At first, I didn't recognize her; she posted under her married name, Gena Lee Hulse. But the photo that accompanied her posts, of a model-perfect gorgeous blonde, was different from most people's Facebook profile photos. Realizing that she seemed familiar, I googled her married name and realized that the rather quiet but compassionate and supportive member of my Thyroid Support group was *the* Gena Lee Nolin of *Baywatch* fame. I realized that she was not trying to call attention to herself, so I didn't mention publicly that we had a celebrity in our midst.

It seemed serendipitous when, a few days later, I received a private message from Gena, asking if she could speak to me. I admit that I didn't really know what to expect. Was she a celebrity diva who wanted free personal advice by phone? I called Gena, and we ended up on the phone for hours, not only talking about thyroid disease, but laughing over shared experiences, life, motherhood, friends, travel . . .we gabbed as if we'd known each other forever. I got to know by phone a funny, sweet, smart, and very down-to-earth wife, mother, and fellow thyroid patient, who had just happened to star on the world's most popular television show!

I was surprised when Gena told me, in her no-nonsense style, that after struggling for nearly two decades with her thyroid symptoms, and finally getting diagnosed, that she felt it was her mission—her obligation—to help raise awareness for thyroid disease, and to help others avoid the fear, the misdiagnosis, and the chronic symptoms that can plague thyroid patients. She felt compelled to do something to help spread the word about thyroid disease and make women—including younger women who might not think they are at risk—aware of this common but often over-looked health challenge.

"I don't want anyone else to feel as alone and scared as I did until I found your page," Gena said.

Gena's passion resonated with me. She articulated her sense of purpose in exactly the same way I did. In that phone call, we quickly decided that we would coauthor a book, a book that would tell Gena's compelling story, educate people about thyroid issues, and hopefully reach an even broader group of women to provide information, empowerment, and peace of mind.

But Gena had another point that resonated with me.

"There seems to be this weird stigma about thyroid disease," said Gena. "No one wants to talk about it, or admit to it. I know dozens of celebrities who have all sorts of thyroid problems—none of them would be caught dead sharing it with the public."

This was true. Celebrity thyroid patients go out of their way to avoid mentioning thyroid conditions, and sometimes even deny diagnoses they'd previously announced.

Gena was adamant. "I want to go public and do whatever I can to raise awareness of thyroid disease. I want young women who are struggling with symptoms to think, 'Hmm . . . Gena Lee Nolin had a thyroid condition, maybe I should get checked out.' I want women to know that it can be hard to get diagnosed, to take yourself seriously, and to get doctors to also take you seriously. And I want women to know that it can strike you whether you're young or old, tall or short, slim or full-figured. And I want them to know that they can live with thyroid disease *and* be sexy!"

It's no secret that thyroid disease is the topic of a variety of cruel jokes. Political correctness says that "fat" jokes are no longer acceptable, so advertisers, sitcoms, and stand-up comics have replaced fat jokes with thyroid jokes. Seinfeld had a famous episode about an old woman with a goiter—the sight of her goiter was so horrifying that Elaine couldn't even look at her in the light of day. Comedian Emo Philips does a bit—which is often shared on Twitter—that goes "I saw a woman wearing a sweatshirt with 'Guess' on it. I said, 'Thyroid problem?'" Advertisers from Dairy Queen to Marriott Hotels have used "thyroid problems" as code for overweight in radio and television ads.

It's no wonder celebrities don't want to reveal their own thyroid problems. "You can never be too young or too thin," goes the saying that Hollywood has adopted wholeheartedly. What celebrity would ever want to reveal a health problem that frequently is associated with weight gain and middle age?

And that's where we come to the "Thyroid Sexy" part of this book.

We've had a Thyroid Sexy community on Facebook, founded by Gena, for several years already. Once in a rare while, someone grumbles about the name . . . they wonder what thyroid has to do with being sexy, or chafe at the idea of thyroid associated with sexiness. But most in the community get it . . . and love it.

Thyroid disease is overlooked, misdiagnosed, brushed aside, and made fun of, and yet it is life-changing. But the image of thyroid disease does not have to be the stereotype of a frumpy, overweight, aging woman—the opposite of what we think of as "sexy." Because, when you're properly diagnosed and treated, and you get your mind, body, and spirit on board, you can be healthy, gorgeous, vital, and yes . . . sexy. Sexy is about how you feel and how you portray yourself to the world, and the energy and passion you bring to your life.

And that's why it's so important that Gena speak out, and why I'm so thrilled to team up with her to write this book. Even as a woman who embodies the concept of "sexy," Gena is so much more. She's a wife, a mother, a businesswoman, an actress, and now an advocate. She is no longer just the beautiful girl in the red swimsuit running down the beach: she's a busy mother, running her children to school, writing, producing, filming, and making her mark on the world in other ways. And now she's hoping that by challenging the stereotype of what thyroid disease looks like, she can make a difference for others.

Sexy is so much more than sex appeal—it's about living life with passion and purpose, feeling comfortable in your own skin, and taking care of yourself. And that's what this book is about. In hearing Gena's story, you will be inspired as you learn how to channel your passion and purpose into your own Thyroid Sexy life.

Mary Shomon
Kensington, Maryland

Introduction

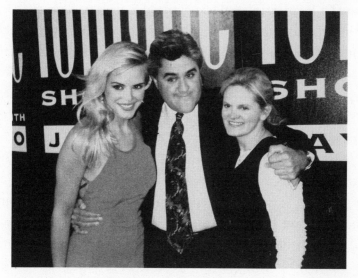

Gena, Jay Leno, and Gena's mom

You're probably thinking, here goes another celebrity book! Which names will she name? What crazy catfights will she reveal? Is she going to offer juicy details of illicit encounters with hunky stars? Are there the required amounts of sex and drugs and rock and roll? Will there at least be a few blockbuster secrets that will end up as tabloid headlines?

The answer is no, no, no, no, and no!

Surprised? Because some people are pretty sure they know me. They assume that the real Gena Lee Nolin is just like the character I played on *Baywatch*, Neely Capshaw. Neely was, for much of her run on the show, a stereotypical "bad girl." She was, to be honest, a pretty vindictive gal, always conniving, quick to seek revenge, and going around trying to steal other women's boyfriends. And then there was the ongoing feud with fellow lifeguard C. J. Parker, played by my friend Pamela Anderson.

Some fans protested when the show's writers changed Neely's character later in the show's run, making her more sympathetic and likable, and, ultimately, having Neely and Mitch—the head lifeguard, played by David Hasselhoff—fall in love and marry. But most *Baywatch* fans remember—and secretly love—the darker, nasty Neely.

I adored playing Neely, especially during her "bad girl" days, because she was my total opposite. Playing against type is an actor's dream. There I was, a happily married "good girl" from Minnesota, running home from the set to make dinner for my husband and learn my lines. I was sorely lacking in any skills at conniving, blackmailing, or meddling, much less stealing other people's men! But it was exhilarating—and, okay, fun!—to play the villain.

But people can't always separate the actor from the character, so, to many people around the world who have seen *Baywatch*, I am Neely.

But the truth is, I'm not Neely, and this is not Neely's story. So, if there isn't going to be intrigue, backstabbing, or steamy story lines, and I'm not planning to blackmail anyone or steal their husband—why read my book?

The answer is simple: because you need to know that you are not alone. And that there is hope.

There was a time I felt alone. I felt alone as I wondered why my body was betraying me on every level, when it seemed everyone else had energy to spare.

I felt alone as I dragged myself out of bed each morning, limbs aching.

I felt alone as I watched my curvy costars on *Baywatch* and wondered how they kept in shape, even as I survived on endless cups of coffee and little else, running up and down the chilly beach fifteen hours a day, watching the weight pile on.

I felt alone at Mommy and Me class, and at the playground, as I struggled to have the energy for even a short play session, and felt like I must be the only mother in the world who could barely lift her precious children.

I felt alone as ever-increasing clumps of my usually long, thick hair clogged my drain.

I felt alone as I looked in the mirror, and staring back at me was a puffy and mottled and almost unrecognizable face.

I felt alone as they rushed me to the hospital, pregnant, trying to figure out why my heart was suddenly beating 200 times a minute, leaving me dizzy, breathless, and faint.

I felt alone as I thought about why, despite having everything a girl could want—a loving husband, precious children, a cozy home, a successful career—I felt like my life was falling apart around me.

I felt alone as I lay sleepless in the middle of the night, so exhausted I could barely move, and convinced that whatever it was that was draining my health would eventually kill me.

I felt alone as I wondered, night after night, "Will I live to see my children grow up?"

Then one day, I finally reached out, connected to the

community of thyroid patients, connected with Mary Shomon, and realized that not only was I not alone, but I could potentially do something to help others never feel alone.

From the bottom of my heart, I hope that you never have to go through the same feelings and fears that I did, and I want to do whatever I can to make sure that you don't. Because what plagued me for two decades and caused the symptoms, the side effects, and the mood swings, was my undiagnosed thyroid condition.

I spent all of my twenties and most of my thirties—years in which I married, had three children, started my television career, appeared on *The Price Is Right,* starred in *Baywatch* and *Sheena,* and moved several times—suffering from undiagnosed and untreated thyroid disease. That's almost twenty years during which I never received a thyroid test or diagnosis. But I did get misdiagnosed with Valley Fever, diabetes, postpartum depression, chronic fatigue syndrome, generalized anxiety disorder, and depression. I've been handed a pharmacy shelfful of various prescription medications that made not even a dent in my symptoms.

And I've even landed in the hospital multiple times with a dangerous heart condition known as atrial fibrillation, which doctors say was likely brought on by my undiagnosed and untreated thyroid problems.

Before my diagnosis, I was told by people I thought were close to me that I was clearly a hypochondriac, that I should see a shrink, consult a hypnotist, visit a Reiki therapist, work out with a trainer, practice yoga, join a church, reduce my stress, or take more vitamins—according to everyone else, pretty much every sort of therapy, supplement, lifestyle, or expert you can think of was the secret solution to my fatigue, mood swings, and weight challenges.

I heard everything but the real answer.

In the end, I needed my symptoms taken seriously. I needed a proper diagnosis. And I needed proper treatment.

Everyone has a story of when they truly hit an emotional wall. In my case, I was in the grocery store in my Los Angeles neighborhood. I had thrown on a pair of shorts and a T-shirt, hair in my usual ponytail and wearing no makeup, as I ran out to pick up some things. Just like any mom. In fact, I was a new mother; my son Spencer had been born just a few weeks earlier. As you can imagine, it took every ounce of energy I had to brush my teeth and put on a clean shirt, instead of going to the store in my PJs! I was standing in the checkout line, holding a sleeping Spencer in his carrier and looking at the covers of *People, Us, Maxim*—covers that featured perfectly coiffed, perfectly posed images of actresses and models—and remembering how not too long before, I'd been in the pages of those same magazines myself. It seemed so long ago already, so very far from my life as a mother and wife.

That's when I heard it . . . loud whispering from two women in line behind me.

"Is that her? Are you sure?" said one woman.

"Definitely!" said the other. "It's her." She snickered.

"She doesn't look anything like she used to," said the first woman.

"Tell me about it," said her friend. "If that's what you have to look like to be on *Baywatch*, I guess anyone can be on the show!"

They both laughed, and I felt their eyes boring a hole in the back of my head.

I felt my whole body tighten. "I will not turn around," I vowed to myself. "I will not say anything. I will keep it together. I won't cry . . ."

I don't even remember paying, or carrying the groceries and Spencer out to the car, or loading the bags and my baby into the car, and fastening his car seat. But I do remember collapsing into the driver's seat and feeling the sobs rising, racking my body. I sat there and sobbed into the steering wheel for an hour. Sobbed because I felt so tired, so spent, so utterly empty inside. Sobbed because a new mother shouldn't have to suffer the indignity of anyone's commenting on how she looked only a few weeks after giving birth. Sobbed because my body, my health, my life—they all seemed to be slipping away. Sobbed because even at a time when I should have been happy, with a new baby, a husband, and a cozy home, I felt adrift, exposed, exhausted, and confused.

The fact is, I've spent the better part of two decades running both toward and away from an image—the Hollywood image—that had come to define me. It's no secret that the entertainment industry is critical of women, demanding perfection in every way. I was expected to have perfect hair, perfect skin, the perfect weight, perfect curves, a perfect family, perfect pregnancies, a perfect body right after pregnancy, and in general, perfect health. In Hollywood, there was always someone willing to cut you down to size and happily broadcast it to the world. Whether it's paparazzi hiding in the bush behind your front door to capture you at your most disheveled, or the photographer snapping shots at a fast-food drive-through, or a radio DJ or TV host berating you for gaining weight, there is an entire industry dedicated to capturing images of, and then tearing down, anyone who has had any sort of celebrity.

We all are running toward and away from these images and expectations that society creates for us—or that we adopt for ourselves. Whether it's our education, job success, physical fitness, being a "Supermom," taking care of elderly parents, or our many other roles, we create these expectations of how we should be, what accomplishments we should be making, and anything less . . . we are often the first to beat ourselves up.

And let's face it . . . others are there to pile on. Whether it's a spouse, family member, coworker, former classmate, or the mother of your child's best friend—you know exactly what I mean. Just when you feel your worst, and are judging yourself harshly, someone comes along who seems determined to make you feel even worse about yourself than you already do.

Who needs it!?

For those of us with thyroid issues, we are trying to feel, look, and do our best—a challenge under the best circumstances—but when you throw in the slow metabolism, thinning hair, exhaustion, and mood changes that come with a thyroid problem, you think, holy Hannah, this is just impossible!

But, as the amazing Audrey Hepburn said, "Nothing is impossible, the word itself says 'I'm possible!'"

When I was in the middle of struggling with my thyroid symptoms, I never thought that a book like *Beautiful Inside and Out* was possible. And now it is!

I think people assume that having thyroid disease means you're older and overweight, but in reality, thyroid disease strikes at all ages and affects all sizes. It's unfortunate that the media, doctors, and the public stereotype thyroid disease as being only about weight gain, when it truly has many faces. You can be thin and have a full head of hair, or exhaustion, or infertility, and be suffering profoundly. In my case, I've gone through all the different stages, from being fit and having healthy hair, to being overweight, puffy, exhausted, depressed, achy, and losing hair by the handful. This is why I feel it's so important to advocate for thyroid patients . . . and to help give thyroid a new and different face.

Beautiful Inside and Out is for the millions of you who have undiagnosed thyroid conditions—like I did, for twenty years . . . maybe even more. Conservative estimates say that at minimum, there are 27 million Americans with thyroid disease, and most of them are women, and most are undiagnosed. When I talk to some of the experts, they say that the actual number of thyroid patients in the United States is actually close to 60 million. That means that one in five Americans probably has a thyroid problem, most of them women who don't even know it. And it's estimated that among my friends in Canada, there are 10 million people with thyroid conditions, and 6 million more in the United Kingdom. Again, the majority are women, and most are undiagnosed.

We are definitely not alone!

That's why it's the perfect time for me to stand up. I'm owning my thyroid disease. I'm publicly and proudly promoting thyroid awareness and doing my best to be a positive voice for other thyroid patients.

I hope that as you read this book, you will soon discover that I'm just like you. Like millions of my fellow thyroid patients, I've run my hands through my hair and noticed how thin and lifeless it felt.

Like so many others with thyroid problems, I've known the frustration of wanting to look my best for a special occasion or event, and the misery of discovering that no matter how hard I exercised, or how little I ate, my body was just not doing what I needed it to do. It didn't make sense. In fact, it seemed almost impossible—how could I eat so little, and work out so much, yet still not lose an ounce? What a helpless feeling. Especially in those times when my job in fact *depended* on my staying in shape.

I've agonized over the health of my unborn babies and cried many days after they were born because I barely had the energy to care for them.

I've had many mornings where I wake up and wonder how I am going to crawl out of bed, get dressed, and make breakfast for my children.

I know the heartbreak of saying "No" when one of the little ones asks to go to the park or my husband wants to have a romantic dinner date, and I simply do not have the energy even to move.

Thyroid disease is not something that affects only our parents and grandparents. It started for me in my twenties. So, if I can help even one person decide, "I'm going to insist on getting my thyroid checked," or if I help someone else understand that things *can and do* get better . . . it will be one of the most important things I can do in this life.

I also want to say that there is light at the end of this tunnel. We can find answers and feel better again, but it's pretty darn hard to do it alone. The good news is, we don't have to.

And that's why this book is so needed. You will find ideas, information, tips, pointers, and advice on how to get properly diagnosed and treated. Believe me, diagnosis is crucial, but holy cow, getting the right kind of treatment after the diagnosis can be a huge challenge in itself.

And *Beautiful Inside and Out* is also for the millions of you who are already diagnosed but know you could feel better, look better, and live better. We have information, resources, and ideas that can help you make sure you are getting the best possible treatment for you.

And because we're turning the image of thyroid on its heels, we'll talk about how to look and feel sassy, beautiful, and sexy. Yes, there I said it, *sexy*!

Because thyroid can be sexy! Sexy is about attitude, and let me tell you, figuring out how to move forward, to live, survive, and thrive despite my thyroid condition has required reaching down deep, and finding my passion and sense of purpose. My goal in *Beautiful Inside and Out* is that you might recognize your own experiences in my story. And if that helps you stand up for yourself with doctors, get a proper diagnosis, find out you have a thyroid condition, and get it properly treated, hooray! Or maybe you'll draw on some extra eyebrows, squeeze into some Spanx, clip on some fake hair, and face the world with your head held high and proud, looking your best! Either way, being smart, confident, and empowered is sexy, and what *Beautiful Inside and Out* is all about!

I welcome you to join me on as we take our journey to wellness. Think of it as if we are sitting together on a cozy couch, over a cup of tea or a glass of wine, and sharing some girl time! Let's get started on living, feeling, and being "thyroid sexy."

Part 1

MY STORY

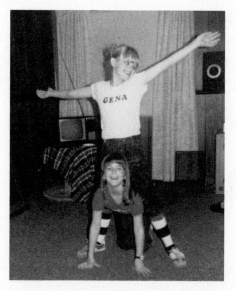

Gena at nine, performing with a friend

1

The Show Must Go On

First say to yourself what would you be;
and then do what you have to do.
—EPICTETUS

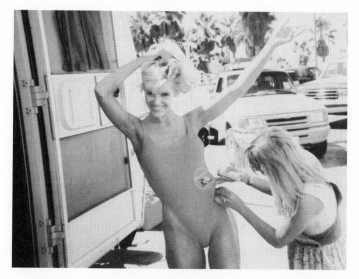

Gena on the Baywatch *set*

It might be a surprise to some people, but I've always been determined, willing to try new things, and open to mastering new skills. That's what landed me my Hollywood career and has helped me face my thyroid challenges. It goes back to my childhood in Duluth, Minnesota, where I grew up with an older brother, Michael, and an older sister, Sheila.

As a toddler, everyone says I was outgoing . . . not the least bit shy. According to Sheila, I was also very determined: "We were looking at old movies my brother put on DVD, and there's Gena at age two, hamming it up for the camera. There's some film of her learning how to skate, she was saying in this determined little voice, 'Don't help me! I'll do it myself!'"

Some of my own earliest memories are of being sick, and the year I was seven was especially tough. I went through weeks of excruciating stomachaches and ended up in the hospital with a ruptured appendix. After the surgery, all I remember is how terrible I felt all the time. My sister also remembers what that year was like: "Gena was always sick, complaining about severe stomachaches, and she barely ate anything. The doctor kept saying it was because she wasn't eating right, but the poor child was hunched over and couldn't even walk. She was so young to be so sick like that."

My mother, Patricia, continued to take me back to the doctor for two years. When I was nine, the symptoms became so bad that they hospitalized me, and that's when they finally discovered what was wrong. My mother explains, "Gena had a mammoth ball of infection in her abdomen. The doctors thought that she must have developed an abscess after her appendix surgery, and it had gotten infected and continued to grow all that year."

Looking back, I remember it was hard to spend so much time in the hospital. But I also remember making friends with other children there. Some had cancer and other serious and chronic diseases. Volunteers brought us books and balloons to cheer us up. I even spent my ninth birthday there. It was a long recuperation from the surgery and left a large, ugly scar on my abdomen that made me reluctant to wear a two-piece swimsuit well into my teenage years.

One of the other major—but far happier—memories of my childhood was putting on shows. I dreamed of being a singer, even though I didn't have the greatest singing voice. But I didn't care. My idol in those days was Olivia Newton-John, and I never tired of singing her songs.

We had a huge deck that overlooked the backyard, and I turned it into my stage. With just an old record player, I recruited my neighborhood friends into an endless series of shows, ordering everyone to sing and dance. I was always the star and MC. I bribed everyone in the neighborhood to come, offering them free Kool-Aid and my mom's homemade cookies if they would sit through my show.

My mother remembers the shows:

> She was as funny and quirky as she is now. She loved to put on those shows, she was very dramatic. The kids would talk, sing, and each one used a jump rope for a microphone. I had made her this gray felt poodle skirt like the one that Olivia Newton-John wore in *Grease,* and she had a T-shirt with her name on it, and that was her entertaining outfit. There she'd be, singing her heart out into a jump rope. Always singing, and finally her dream came true, she went to an Olivia Newton-John concert, and of course, she wore her poodle skirt!

Though I was close to my father when I was little, he was abusive. When I was eleven, my world as I knew it fell apart when my mom put Sheila, Michael, and me in the car, and in the middle of the night, we moved away from Duluth. We lived in Colorado for a while, and then moved back to Minnesota where my grandmother lived. From that point onward, I didn't have much to do with my father, and sadly, our relationship was strained from there on out.

It was hard. My mother was worried about making ends meet, I didn't have a father, and I was the youngest. I always put on a brave, tough exterior, but inside, I felt confused about where I fit.

When onstage, making people smile or laugh, I could feel at peace during a time when everything else felt complicated. When I stood on our backyard stage, the world always felt right.

We ended up moving to Las Vegas, and that's where I attended high school.

Through my early teens, I felt like an ugly duckling—tall, gawky, and awkward. It's funny to say now, but I avoided wearing swimsuits. There I was, doing whatever I could to not have to wear a swimsuit, and I ended up making my living in one!

When I was around sixteen, I lost my baby pudge and started to become interested in clothes. I tried to be stylish, even though we were on a tight budget. My friend Ann's mother was a great seamstress, and she helped us make some great outfits from Vogue patterns.

My mom remembers what it was like.

Gena had her own style. She's never been "Oh, I have to have this or that style." She would just get a feel for what she thought was cool and different, and try things out. And sure enough, if she wore something, the other girls would often follow her style. Gena was also someone who wanted to bring people together and create a community. She told me that everyone at high school was so uptight and stressed. So I helped her start a massage class in her high school. And it wasn't too long before they were all working on each other's backs!

I started to get some attention from boys, but truthfully . . . I felt too shy to do much about it.

I did meet a gorgeous young junior fireman, Steve, who was new on the force. He asked Mom if he could drop by sometime to say hello to me. The day he decided to come by with another fire-fighter buddy, I heard him at the door. I'll let Mom tell the rest of the story: "Gena ran to her bathroom. 'Mom! I don't want him to see me!' She was dressed in a pair of shorts and a T-shirt, but she put on her bathrobe over her clothes and put on a green mud mask, with a towel on her hair, and then came out to say hello to Steve the fireman. She said, 'Oh, hi! I was just getting out of the tub!'"

My mom has since told me that she always wondered why I did that. The truth is, I had a major crush on Steve . . . he was smart, funny, handsome, just a few years older than me, and he had a cute car—everything a girl could want! But I wasn't feeling my best that day. I had a big zit that had popped up, and I was just wearing my hanging-out clothes, and so I figured, better to look like I just got out of the shower. It made sense to me, but according to Mom, they didn't care. "Steve and his pal were still totally smitten with her, despite her robe and towel disguise! She did end up going out with Steve for a while."

Something unusual started to happen. I noticed that wherever I went, people would stop and ask me, "Are you a movie star?" "Are you a model?" It was so embarrassing. I remember one time, walking through a store, and this person came up to Mom and me and asked me if I was an actress. "Isn't that dumb?" I asked Mom.

Even with my history of putting on shows and early dreams of being a singer, the thought of going into entertainment never crossed my mind. But many people assumed I was already "in the business" as a teenager.

When I was sixteen, my brother told me that I was "sort of cute." (Brothers are so funny!) Michael suggested that we send some pictures in to a Ford Models Look of the Year contest that he'd seen written up in the newspaper. He had me put on a cute blouse, and he took the pictures himself at our apartment, and we sent them in to the contest.

Next thing I knew, I had a phone call from Katie Ford herself, in New York City. Holy Toledo! I'd won the regional competition, up against forty other girls. I was still reluctant to get into modeling, though.

When I was seventeen, my mother and I were at the mall one day, and an older guy came up and started talking to us. Mom remembers that day:

He was my age, and I'm thinking, "Okay, so what do *you* want, what's your angle?" He was talking about the Miss Las Vegas for Jaycees pageant. I didn't know if he was on the up-and-up, or just trying to hit on Gena. So I got his card, then called and found out more, and it turned out that it was legitimate. I asked Gena if it was something she might want to do; after all, it could be kind of fun. She decided to do it, so she borrowed some cool black leather pants—she had to have a pants outfit and a dress outfit—and borrowed a blue dress, and we went to Payless and bought her royal blue matching shoes. She competed against sixty-four contestants, and she was first place for the tall division. She won a photo shoot in New York, and a scholarship to Barbizon in New York City. After two days at Barbizon, the owner asked Gena to compete for the Miss Barbizon title. So there's Gena, with no experience, and she walked away the winner . . . Miss Barbizon.

It felt as if modeling was choosing me, instead of the other way around. So, at eighteen, I was off to spend three months in New York. I didn't know a soul and was somewhat nervous at first about being in the city. The first few weeks, I spent so much money on cabs, because I was afraid to use the subway. But everyone I met told me that real New Yorkers took the subway, so I finally got up the nerve. And at that point, I became fearless and explored everything—I went to all the museums, I took the Staten Island Ferry, walked in Central Park. I was also doing some modeling, including for J Crew.

The other models and I would go to a little pub at the end of our street in Chelsea. That's when I met actor Timothy Hutton, who invited me to come see the Broadway play *Love Letters*. We became friends, and I would go to his house in SoHo for his amazing dinner parties. I met the quintessential New Yorker, Woody Allen, and Tim Hutton even let me hold his Oscar from the film *Ordinary People* . . . so exciting!

In the end, the New York agency decided that my look was not a good fit for the East Coast, which was really into the brunette, exotic, Cindy Crawford look in those days. And there I was, the blond, blue-eyed, beachy, California girl-next-door type. So back to Las Vegas I went.

After high school, my friend Alicia and I decided to move to Los Angeles. She was an aspiring model and actress, and she always wanted to make it big in Hollywood. At that point, I had done the little bit of modeling, but otherwise, I didn't really know what I wanted to do. However, I knew that whatever I was going to do, it was going to be in California! Even as a young girl putting on my shows, I knew L.A. was magic, and I had to go.

So we packed up my Toyota Tercel and moved to L.A. We found a little studio apartment, and we ran a piece of masking tape down the middle to split up our living space.

I liked my new life in Los Angeles. I had my little car. I had outfitted the cozy apartment with a beachy sofa and chair I loved, and a television. I got little doodads at the Pick and Save to spiff up the apartment. I was nineteen, and I was creating a life for myself.

For work, I had a retail job at Broadway Southwest—now Macy's—at the Beverly Center in Beverly Hills, and worked as a cocktail waitress at the restaurant Mezzaluna. I also enrolled at Santa Monica College to take some courses while I was working the two jobs.

But I needed to decide on a more serious occupation. I didn't want to be a cocktail waitress or work retail forever. I looked into being a flight attendant, and I thought about physical therapy . . . I wanted to move into a service-oriented career.

I watched Alicia go to audition after audition, but I never really thought about getting into the business. What we did do, for extra money, were some promotional modeling jobs—trade shows, car shows, that sort of thing. A friend from those days has called Alicia and me "the Laverne and Shirley of promotional modeling."

We were young, and on our own for the first time, yet I started to notice that there were many days when I was so completely exhausted I could barely make it through the day. It surprised me; as an active, healthy young woman, I expected to be able to keep up with anything life was throwing at me at the time—but I would find myself needing a nap before going out at night, or sleeping in on the weekends. I always seemed to be more tired than Alicia and the other women my age. I tried to chalk it up to working too hard at my various jobs, but all my friends were also working multiple jobs, but they had the energy to also enjoy the L.A. nightlife, work out, and hit the beach on weekends. With my constant exhaustion, I could barely drag myself from job to job . . . I had this feeling something more was wrong, but I didn't know even where to start finding out what was going on.

Alicia and I were sent to Las Vegas for a promotional modeling job at a film production trade show. I was standing around handing out literature at the show when I met Greg Fahlman, who ran a film production company in Canada and was attending the conference. He came over to our table, and we started talking. He was a cute guy, older than me by at least ten years, but he was smart and funny, and throwing out these hilarious one-liners. I felt an immediate connection. He asked me to have lunch with him, and I said yes. After he left, I told Alicia, "He's not going to come back." But secretly, I was hoping he would. Sure enough, five minutes before my break, he showed up, and we went to have lunch. It was unbelievable. We hit it off and had a strong bond from the start.

Greg also remembers that night. "She seemed like a lovely girl. I asked if she had plans for dinner that evening, and she said she had a friend with her, so why not, I invited them both out to dinner! From there, we went out that evening, hit a few fun parties. The next weekend I flew to Los Angeles, and we had a long-distance relationship—me in Canada, and Gena in Los Angeles—and visiting each other back and forth, for two years."

After two years, Greg decided to move to Los Angeles, and that's when things got serious. It was one of those things—when you meet someone and you just know that you're going to have something very special with that person—that kind of connection. Sometimes I wonder if part of the attraction was his age—he was about eleven years older, and he was very protective of me. I hadn't felt a man's protection since my father left a decade earlier. With Greg, I felt very taken care of.

We married, had a beautiful wedding, and moved in together, very much in love. He was so smart and intense, but at the same time, he was protective, and he had my back. I felt very safe.

Greg saw a potential in me that I didn't even see myself. I think from the start, he envisioned an entertainment career for me, so he was on the lookout for opportunities.

I still hadn't thought about acting, but Greg said that we should at least take some photographs. He sent my head shots off, and I got signed with a modeling agency and started to do some modeling jobs.

Then came a day that completely changed my life. I'll let Greg tell the story: "I'd read somewhere that one of the gals on *The Price Is Right*—Dian Parkinson—was leaving the show, and they were looking for a replacement. Gena looked very much like a younger version of Dian, so we mailed off her photos to the executive producer. Gena was one of the last girls they saw, out of more than a thousand girls. They invited her in for a tryout."

I'd never been on television before. I went in for a twenty-minute audition and had to show a desk, wearing a bathing suit. (Seriously. How awkward was that?) After that first audition, they called back and had me do six test shows with the rest of the cast. I decided I should just follow the lead of the other women who had been there forever, do my best, and not ruffle any feathers.

I was on pins and needles, waiting to find out, talking to every girlfriend, every family member: "Will they pick me? Will they pick me?" They were all saying, "Enough already. If you get it, you get it." When they called, I was in Canada, visiting friends. In the end, after seeing 1,300 girls for the spot, they picked me.

Greg called it the "best part-time job in the world," and it was.

I enjoyed the camaraderie on the set of *The Price Is Right*; the crew parties and birthday celebrations had a family feeling. Apparently I was doing a good job. One of the show's producers, Phillip Rossi, even told *People* magazine, "Nolin can bring energy to standing next to a refrigerator." (Hey, I'll take the compliment!)

Bob Barker was so good to me, and a joy to work with. I also became close friends with one of the original Barker's Beauties, Holly Hallstrom. She was a strong, opinionated woman, and became not only a friend but a mentor to me. She had a gorgeous house in Laurel Canyon, and used to invite me over to have tea. We shared a love of decorating, and she had impeccable taste.

With my first paycheck from *The Price Is Right*, I bought myself a new Singer sewing machine so I could make curtains, pillows, place mats . . . you name it, I'd sew it. I wanted to create that same cozy feeling in our little apartment that I got in Holly's house!

I didn't have an agent when I landed *The Price Is Right*, but the minute I got that job, the William Morris Agency called. And after I signed with them, it was wild—I went from 0 to 60 in terms of opportunities. All of a sudden, I was being asked to make appearances, shoot ads, and go to events.

A few months into my work on *The Price Is Right*, I received a call to audition for *The Bold and the Beautiful*. I still couldn't envision myself as an actress. I had no lines on *The Price Is Right*. I had never even seen a script!

I didn't end up getting the big part on *The Bold and the Beautiful*, but I was cast as a model named Sandra who didn't say much. I figured it was a sign that I'd better stick to showing microwave ovens and fabulous new refrigerator-freezers!

One day I got a call from my agent. The show *Baywatch* wanted me to come in and read for them. *Baywatch*. Which at the time had an audience of *one billion fans* in 110 countries.

Meanwhile, my claim to fame was smiling and looking cute while I pointed at appliances. I didn't want to go, and couldn't imagine how I would get a part like this, with no acting experience.

I also knew it was a show about lifeguards, which meant I'd have to spend most of my time in a swimsuit. That was also a pretty daunting thought, to be honest, as I was already starting to notice that my metabolism was not what it had been during my teenage years. So Greg really had to push me to try out for the part. He remembers, "The first step in the audition was a 6:30 a.m. swim, and Gena was saying 'No, I'm not going to do this!' I told her that she absolutely had to do it, and I drove her to the pool for the swim audition. Some of the women trying out weren't water savvy, but Gena was athletic and a strong swimmer. She also worked particularly hard to learn the audition lines."

I really studied the lines, determined to do my best. I ended up reading with different producers, including David Hasselhoff, and put my entire heart into it! I didn't care if I looked like a fool or overacted, I just did it. I clicked right away with Hassel—everyone calls him that. He's charismatic and has a huge personality, and it was easy to act with him.

They had me in for a callback, and this time they said it was a screen test. So I was even more nervous than usual. The set was filled with a huge crew, many cast members, and all sorts of cameras. I decided to go for it. There I was, acting my heart out, and I looked up and noticed that David was waving a red lifeguard can at me. I was thinking, "Why is David being a jerk with the can when I'm in the middle of the audition of my life?!"

"Read it!" people started yelling to me.

Written on the lifeguard can were the words *You've got the part!*

I just stood there, dumbstruck.

All of a sudden, everyone was cheering, and jumping up and down. The whole screen test was a setup, because they'd already decided to cast me in the part of Neely Capshaw.

Entertainment Tonight was there, and they were in on the prank and filmed the whole thing, including my surprised reaction at learning that I had the job. They ran the segment that evening.

Greg explains how thrilling it was:

That was the moment our lives changed forever. People don't realize, but *Baywatch* was a cultural phenomenon at the time— and Gena's getting a starring role on the show catapulted her into an entirely new life for both of us. The night she got the part, she was on *Entertainment Tonight,* and the very next day she was on a plane to the Bahamas for a promotional shoot, and it was in all the papers by end of the week. From that point, the paparazzi started following her everywhere.

Meanwhile, I had to quickly get into the rhythm of being an actress. And it was tough!

I was learning how to act as I went along, but Neely was a fun character to play. She was always into something, on pills, drunk, chasing every guy around—she was everything I wasn't. I used to say that I had to conjure up my worst PMS moods in order to give her the right attitude. I was able to let go and be rotten, rant and rave, and then come home and sew or just chill. She was a blast to play once I got the hang of it!

In addition to learning acting on the job, the physical demands were challenging. As Hassel used to say, "The water is cold, the sand is hot, and the days are very long." So true.

I had to wake up before 4 a.m. and be on the set and in the makeup chair by 4:30 a.m. There were days when it was so difficult to drag myself out of bed, but I always did. Filming began at sunrise, and then it was a day filled with all that famous running up and down the beach, jumping off moving boats, back in hair and makeup again, more running, and in between, reading and learning lines. Sometimes we didn't wrap until as late as 7 p.m.

I was also doing double duty for a while. Even though I'd gotten *Baywatch*, I didn't want to leave *The Price Is Right*, so, for a few months I kept both jobs going. I told Bob Barker that I wasn't sure I was going to make it with the acting. Bob laughed, and said, "There's no way you're coming back, kid. Go out there and be the star you are!" I'll never forget those words.

I did keep it going for a while—working for *Baywatch*, and

then racing back to shoot *The Price Is Right*. But eventually I realized I couldn't do it anymore. It wasn't fair to either show, and I was starting to get some popularity on *Baywatch*, and they were making a bigger deal about my character. Pamela Anderson was becoming more famous than ever—she'd just married Tommy Lee—and our show was in the press every day . . . *Entertainment Tonight*, *Hard Copy*, and such. So I left *The Price Is Right* and committed myself to *Baywatch*.

On the set, in between all the hair, makeup, and filming, I barely sat down and hardly had time to grab a cup of coffee, much less to eat properly. Even though I was pin thin in those days, I was so worried about how I looked in the swimsuit that I didn't want to eat anyway. I remember the other girls on *Baywatch* eating, and I was getting by on half a bagel and a juice every day. I was thinking, *Oh my gosh, how can they do that?*

I was working sixty-hour weeks on *Baywatch*, I was also being asked to do more interviews, television commercials, magazine ads, and personal appearances, so I was putting in close to ninety hours a week. I blamed the intense schedule and the physicality of being on *Baywatch* for the way I felt, but truth be told, every day I was more and more exhausted.

A strange numbness—beyond fatigue, beyond anything I'd ever experienced—set in. I felt like I was in a fog, just going through the motions.

There I was in Hollywood, with my husband, on a successful television show, living a life most actresses can only dream about, but I was finding it increasingly difficult to enjoy what was happening. I couldn't figure out why I was tired all the time. I wanted to have the energy that others seemed to have so effortlessly. And despite a steady stream of people in my life—agents, producers, actors, cast, friends—I still felt lonely, like I should have been enjoying it more.

I think I also felt guilty and unworthy of the success. I'd seen my mother, brother, and sister struggle. I knew there were actors far more talented than me, who had spent years studying acting and who were barely getting by, relegated to waiting tables . . . I'd do my ten lines, put on a swimsuit, run down the beach, and make a lot of money. It seemed unfair.

There was a never-ending list of parties I was expected to attend, but I was so exhausted all the time, I rarely wanted to go. My mother was surprised: "Her agent would say so-and-so will be there, and it's a good idea for you to make a showing. But Gena just did not want to go. She was always so tired. She just wanted to stay home and sleep."

While I was doing *Baywatch*, Greg was acting as my manager. As a take-charge type of person, he was taking the phone calls, shielding me, and protecting me business-wise, but I still felt like I was always working, all the time. And outside of working, I felt so incredibly tired.

The long days, early hours, and all that running—plus the other responsibilities—were taking a toll. I didn't want to complain, because who in her right mind complains about being on a hit television show? But the producers could see that I was getting run-down, so they made an appointment for me to see a doctor.

I now suspect that this was the beginning of my long battle with undiagnosed thyroid disease, but at that time, the doctor didn't do any blood tests. Instead, he decided that I was suffering from some depression, so he prescribed an antidepressant. I took the pills, but, not surprisingly, they didn't help. I was still completely spent and struggling to keep up with my *Baywatch* schedule.

Meanwhile, the show was continuing to become more popular, and the paparazzi and entertainment shows never let up. Every night, there was a blurb, "Pamela has been seen here," or "Gena has been seen there." One day, I looked out my door, and there was actually a guy up in the trees, shooting pictures of me as I walked out the door. It was bizarre. It was as if they could always find me, no matter what. I would go for a walk in Laurel Canyon with my dogs—I loved it there—and even though I hadn't told a soul I was going, almost every time I went, up popped a photographer!

On the *Baywatch* set at the beach, there was always a horde of paparazzi every morning from sunrise until we stopped for the day. They were trying to get shots of anything, but the more unflattering the image, the better. We had a phone booth near the lifeguard tower—and those were the days before cell phones—so we all used that phone. I remember one day, Yasmine Bleeth was using the phone and she scratched her nose. The next week, a tabloid published a photo with the headline "Yasmine Bleeth Picking Her Nose." It was ridiculous! As soon as you left your trailer, you had to be on guard. I pretty much always wore a robe as soon as I left the trailer, because they were just waiting to catch you at your worst. It was a public beach, so it was crazy. And whenever Pam Anderson was filming, Tommy Lee often came along, and that meant there were even more paparazzi than usual.

Still, it wasn't all exhaustion and paparazzi.

One of the best parts of working on *Baywatch* was how wonderfully I got along with Hassel. When he walked into a room, everyone noticed. He has that big personality, and the voice, which I loved. From the start, he got me to open up, and relax, to have fun with it.

He would compliment me so respectfully . . . telling me I was smart, prepared, or that I looked beautiful. I had come from showing microwave ovens and Tupperware on *The Price Is Right,* and now I was on the number one show in the world, and this guy who was larger than life, who was acting before I was born, was giving me compliments . . . compliments I very much needed at the time. He also often told me how impressed he was at how hard I worked to study my lines.

And I did. I couldn't understand actors who came to set without knowing their lines. I always knew my lines and took my job very seriously. Hey, it wasn't Shakespeare, but it was my job, and I wanted to do it well.

He appreciated that. Hassel has a photographic memory and could literally flip through the pages and shoot a scene. I've never seen anything like it.

There were good days and bad days, but throughout that first season, I kept at it, getting to the set before sunrise and working long days, and then collapsing in exhaustion at home, until we finally wrapped my first season at the end of 1995.

To be honest, the wrap party was by far my favorite day on the show. It was so much fun to have the writers, crew, and cast together in one place. Everyone was relaxed, no deadlines, and we were able to really kick back and enjoy ourselves. I felt relieved to know I was going to have a break.

That Christmas, I went home to Minnesota and spent the holidays with my family. It was a good reality check to be around my family. But right after Christmas, I had a call from *The Tonight Show,* and they wanted to fly me in to be on the show as a last-minute replacement for someone who couldn't make it.

I really didn't want to go. I was on my break with my family, it was so cozy, and I didn't want to leave. But you don't say no to Jay Leno. I had already been on the show a few times and had a great rapport and connection with Jay, whether it was doing an interview or the funny skits we would do together.

But it was Christmas week. So I said, "If you're going to make me leave home at the holidays, then you have to fly my entire family out too. It's a package deal." And Jay agreed. We were all so jazzed! So we packed up Grandma Marie, Mom, Greg, and me, and we all flew to L.A. and had a great time. I was so thrilled to have them all there, and I don't think my grandma could have been any prouder! How often do you get to bring your grandma to the set of her favorite TV show?

Meanwhile, I was back to shooting my second season of *Baywatch*, and in the meantime, also shooting a lot of television commercials. They were writing Neely into more story lines and giving her more dialogue, so I had more reading and studying to do, but I had gotten a better handle on the overall routine.

Still, my exhaustion was getting progressively worse, and the antidepressant hadn't helped a bit. And on top of it all, I had a case of "baby on the brain." All I could think about was how much I wanted to just stay home, have a baby, and not live this crazy life. Greg and I had been married for four years by then, and even though I was constantly on the run, my idea of heaven was to be home with a baby, sewing, and keeping house. (The way I see it, I'd have been a perfect doctor's wife!) To me, that felt like a real life, and my constant motion from sets to shoots and jetting around, well, that didn't feel real at all.

Greg didn't understand at first why I wanted to have a baby:

I had been married and had two children before Gena and I were married. So initially when she said she wanted a child I thought she was crazy, we should wait. But family was number one to Gena, and she was clear that she would much rather have a strong and happy family than the success and fame. She enjoyed being in entertainment, but at the end of the day, her definition of success was based on having a happy family. Because she came from a fractured family, a healthy, happy family gave her the sense of security she craved.

Finally Greg agreed we could start trying. Meanwhile, I had made a decision. I went in to see the show's producers and told them I wanted to quit the show, that I couldn't handle another season given my exhaustion. I told them that given the choice of my health or being famous, I picked my health.

They were horrified because they felt Neely had become a key character on the show and I couldn't be replaced. "We can't let you go because Neely is an important part of story line."

They thought I was just playing them for more money, but I really did want to leave, and wanted to get out of my contract, which I'd signed for five years. They kept telling me my character was popular. When they finally realized I was serious, they decided they needed a way to help encourage me to stay. So they talked me out of leaving and talked me into seeing a hypnotist, of all things. A flippin' hypnotist?! I laughed and cried then laughed again because they were actually serious! I went along with it, and it actually helped me relax, plus I got a raise! Who would have thought?

Meanwhile, I still had baby on the brain, and I figured out that if I timed the pregnancy right, I could work it out so I didn't have to miss too much time on *Baywatch*. I figured out exactly when to get pregnant, and surprise, I got pregnant the first time we tried.

I didn't tell anyone. I waited until we wrapped the season, and then I told everyone and was able to relax a bit.

Along the way, I found out we were having a boy. It was a memorable day because Grandma and Mom—all three generations of us—were there at the ultrasound to get that first glimpse of my precious first son.

One of the key people who came into my life during this time was my friend Janell. I love how Janell tells the story of how we met:

> I had just moved to L.A. from Edmonton. There was a woman in Edmonton whose husband was friends with Greg, Gena's husband. At that time, Gena was on *Baywatch*, and so I called, and ended up on the phone with Gena for two hours . . . we just clicked. She invited me over, and we had a potluck dinner. I was telling her that I was a Sagittarius and things sometimes come out of my mouth the wrong way.
>
> Gena said, "No way! Me too!"
>
> I asked her if she walks into walls right in front of her.
>
> "All the time!" she said. "When's your birthday?"
>
> When I told her it was November 29th, she started laughing, because it was her birthday too. A friendship was born.

Janell and I are so similar, though we are like night and day in some ways. For example, Janell is totally a party girl. I'll be begging her to stay home and watch a movie, have a glass of wine, and curl up on the couch, and she's always itching to go to the latest event or restaurant or hotspot. But she was a true friend to me throughout the pregnancy, and has been ever since.

Pregnancy was on the one hand joyous but at the same time hard. The idea of becoming a mother for the first time was overwhelming. And physically, I knew that I had to be return to the show soon after the baby arrived, so I was worried about weight gain.

With Spencer I craved tangerine juice—I would go to the farmer's market and drink a gallon of tangerine juice. One month, I packed on fifteen pounds between two visits, and the doctor said, "What are you doing?" I told him about the juice, and he told me I needed to cut it out!

So I became much more careful about what I ate. Even so, I gained forty pounds with Spence. In the end, my body just did what it was going to do.

At one point, I was far along in the pregnancy, big as a barrel, and majorly craving a burger. So I went to the drive-through at McDonald's and got a Big Mac. I noticed some paparazzi taking photos, but didn't think much of it. Until the next day, when I was driving in the car, and heard on the radio "Tonight, on *Hard Copy*, *Baywatch* babe Gena Lee Nolin scarfing down a Big Mac." I watched the show, and let's just say it was not flattering. There was the footage of me, in my car in the parking lot, eating my Big Mac.

Everyone wanted pictures or film of the big, fat, pregnant *Baywatch* babe. I spent a lot of time late in my pregnancy hiding out, avoiding any more of those scenes.

My mother was there for Spencer's birth. Mom is a massage therapist, yoga teacher, and doula, so she was the best person to help coach me through. My mom had always wanted me to try to have a natural childbirth, but when I went into labor, I quickly realized it was not going to happen. Here's how my mom remembers it: "Gena was not happy. She said, 'Mother, I don't know how you did this, I'm going crazy!' I was encouraging her to go for an unmedicated birth—helping her breathe and focus. But she decided she really needed the epidural. She said, 'If I don't get some medication, I'm going to jump out of this window and land in front of Jerry's Deli!' That was the deli right next to the hospital. She got her epidural."

Spencer was born June 3, 1997, and he was a beautiful, good baby, and the joy of my life.

One of the best parts of having Spencer, though, was how close I felt to my mother. I was overwhelmed with love for Mom, realizing that she had done this at such a young age, and had three young children, and so much of it she did alone. I would call her, and say "How did you do this?" She was very much there for me.

I learned how patient a mother has to be. Before you have kids, you're on an airplane, and you hear a child screaming, and think "Can't you shut your kid up?" But once you become a mother, it's like you've gotten a patience transfusion! I gained a new appreciation for her. I think of how she grew as a woman, and I felt inspired.

But symptoms hit me hard after he was born. I thought *Baywatch* was exhausting, but *nothing* prepared me for how I felt after Spencer's birth! I was in my early twenties, physically fit, and, maybe I was naive, but to be honest, I expected to bounce back quickly. Instead, in those early weeks, I was an exhausted, fuzzy-brained, depressed, bloated mess. I kept finding myself crying. This was not like me.

Meanwhile, I was having nightmares that I might never get in good enough shape to put on "the red suit" again for *Baywatch*. When I got back into exercising, it was a shocker to me how my body was *not* cooperating. It was like, "Yoo-hoo, Gena, I am NOT listening to you!" no matter what I did. I had to throw myself fully into working out, and it was grueling. There were tears, but I was determined and motivated, because my physical fitness was my livelihood and my trademark, so I was going to have to get back into that suit. I had personal trainers coming to the house, I was climbing hills, biking, doing everything I could. I was lunging, squatting, and exercising like nobody's business, and eating almost nothing. I was not a model of healthy behavior, looking back, but at the time, it seemed like keeping my job depended on it, and I was finally able to drop the baby weight and get in shape.

While I was still on maternity leave, I went over to the *Baywatch* set with Spencer. I still remember, I had on Guess jeans overalls—I lived in those when I was pregnant—and had Spencer in a BabyBjörn. Everyone fell in love with him and his chubby cheeks. And Hassel got excited, deciding on the spot that he had to write a baby for me into the story line. He decided that our characters should marry, and that I should have a baby from my ex. He was going to turn nasty Neely into a good girl. (Shoot! I actually really loved being the bad girl!)

Before I went back to work, *Access Hollywood*, *InStyle*, *Extra*, and *Entertainment Tonight* all came to do "Gena and her new baby" pieces. I was so used to putting on the Hollywood Gena face—the fake part of me—and so I did my makeup and hair, tidied the house, put an adorable outfit on Spencer, and made it all look perfect. But the night before each of these interviews, I would cry, doubting what I was doing, questioning whether I was a good mother, and wondering why I was so exhausted and depressed. When the cameras rolled, though, I always made it seem perfect.

Awhile after Spence was born, my mom decided to go back home to her yoga studio, but I really needed her. She worked it out to have some other folks take over the studio, she rented out her house, and came back to L.A. I went back to work two months after Spencer was born, and my mom and Spencer were on set every day until sunset.

While my mother was caring for Spencer, I was back to the long hours and feeling worse than ever. Doing *Baywatch* in the days before Spence seemed easy in comparison to how I felt now. Again, looking back, I can now see that I was struggling with my thyroid, especially after having had a baby, but I didn't know.

The days were so incredibly long. I had to become a super-hero woman on set, a sex symbol with perfect hair and perfect makeup, appearing to everyone on site that I was happy-go-lucky, without a care in the world. Meanwhile, inside, I was feeling more exhausted than ever before.

Did Pam Anderson feel this way? She was a new mother, too. But she seemed able to keep up with all the filming and still have energy to party and live a glamorous celebrity life. Some of the other actors actually came to the set in the morning, directly from all-night parties. How could they do that and still work?

I barely had time to be with my baby, and it seemed as if the only time we had together was his nightly bath, after I got home from the set.

I just wanted to feel normal and happy like other moms. I was twenty-five years old, yet I felt fifty.

I went back to the doctor, told him that I was dragging myself around in a constant state of exhaustion, and feeling down in the dumps. Again, he didn't run any blood tests. He decided that this time, I was suffering from postpartum depression. He put me back on antidepressants just around the time I stopped breast-feeding.

I think my complaints just went in one ear and out the other. I was hurt, but I understood. I felt inadequate, helpless, and hopeless. I would complain to my girlfriends, but they quickly got tired of my complaints. I remember one night, getting together for drinks, and when I started to talk, one friend said, "Gena, can we please *not* talk about your not feeling well today?"

People wrote me off—and I felt like I was a hypochondriac. Even some family members lost patience. I remember one person saying to me, "Okay, Gena, what's next? Every time we see you, you're complaining about something new."

I started to believe some of what they were saying—maybe I was crazy, maybe it was in my head.

I went to a psychiatrist, and he said I didn't have any mental health issues . . . I was just anxious because I clearly didn't feel well.

I never talked about my health with anyone on set. I wasn't one to complain at work.

I remember when I was back on the set, I had a volleyball scene on the beach with Carmen Electra, Donna D'errico, and Pam Anderson, and I was in the suit, thinking, "Uh-oh!" By that point, I had managed to lose as much weight as I could—not in a healthy way—but I felt intimidated because I definitely didn't measure up to the other girls. Donna's son was six. And even though Pam had had a baby recently, she was a tough act to follow. She's got a rocking body—gifted, frankly—and she bounces right back. (I've also always felt like a moose next to her. I've always been a big girl; I'm big-boned, and at five foot nine, I tower over Pam.)

At the same time, though, there was this little voice inside—kind of a maternal instinct kicking in—that said, "Screw it! You look okay, don't be too hard on yourself!" But it was so hard to listen to that little voice, being on set with all these women who looked so perfect.

In addition to the show, when Spencer was just nine weeks old, we filmed a special *Baywatch* episode. It was going to be the wedding of Mitch—played by David Hasselhoff—and Neely. The whole film was going to take place on a cruise to Alaska. It was a big deal at the time; they even put out Neely and Mitch Barbie dolls.

Mom agreed to go with me, and we flew with Spence to Vancouver, where the cruise was leaving. I was still a bit heavier than I wanted to be, but luckily, I had only one scene in a bathing suit. Otherwise, I was clothed, and I could have a stand-in or body double if I needed it.

Alaska was one of the most beautiful places I'd ever been. And the filming went well. Neely and Mitch got married. Hassel even put Spencer in a scene where he sings him to sleep. My little boy looked like an angel. The only catch? I had a baby girl in the story line, so Mr. Spencer was baby Ashley—dressed in girly baby clothes. (He still cringes about it!)

I continued on for a while, but I was increasingly exhausted. I'd lost my passion and energy for the show. I went back to the producers and asked them to let me out of the contract, and they finally agreed. We had an understanding and respectful departure, and they hired another actress to play out Neely's role. (A few years later, when they did a special *Baywatch* Hawaii film that included Neely, they asked me to come back and be part of that film, and I gladly accepted.)

I walked away from a starring role on a hit television show because I wanted to be a mother to my son. I didn't have the energy to do both, and I still didn't understand why.

2

Married with Children

Love is all we have, the only way that each can help the other.

—EURIPIDES

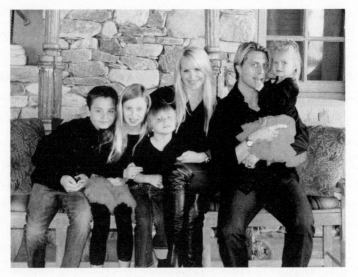

Gena and family

Life after *Baywatch* was very much family oriented. Greg and I started spending time in Scottsdale, Arizona, where he had family. I had never been there before but fell in love with the area . . . it felt immediately like home. Scottsdale was just a quick plane ride to L.A., but it was a world apart. I liked the lifestyle there; it was clean and great for raising a family. I saw children riding their bicycles around the neighborhood, something that couldn't happen in my busy Los Angeles neighborhood. I felt like I could finally breathe. So we decided to make that our primary home, and we bought a house.

I spent a lot of time being a homemaker—fixing up our new house and taking care of Spence.

Going from *Baywatch* to being a stay-at-home mom was wonderful—Spencer and I got into a rhythm and transitioned beautifully. I enjoyed being at home and being a homemaker far more than the hustle and bustle. I could be myself.

At the same time, I wondered if being myself was enough. What did people think of the new me? Did they judge me for leaving Hollywood? Was I a good enough mother?

I also struggled to make new friends. Back in Los Angeles, I always had friends, not to mention the ever-present entourage of photographers, media, colleagues, and fans. Here I was on my own.

I was trying to make friends and figure out how to fit into the Scottsdale mom scene, and at first, I wasn't doing a very good job of it. As a toddler, Spencer was very energetic. He would run around at get-togethers with other children. I later learned that he had ADD, but at that time, I just thought he was high-spirited. At one playgroup, they pulled me aside and said, "Your son is just running around too much, and freaking the other kids out, and we need you to leave."

Kicked out of a playgroup! Excuse me? My mama lion came out and all I could think was that they could take their playgroup and stick it where the sun don't shine!

I was also surprised to discover that after quitting *Baywatch*, I was more exhausted than ever before. I woke up every day exhausted—even after a full night's sleep—and struggled with constant headaches and body pain. I had thought leaving the show was going to help, but it felt like my symptoms were getting worse every day.

One doctor I saw decided that I probably had Valley Fever—a flulike fungal infection, common in some parts of Arizona and other areas of the Southwest—that causes fatigue, headaches, muscle pain, and joint pain. I had those symptoms, so he ran a test, but it came back negative.

A few weeks later, I saw that same doctor, and I remember it was a Friday afternoon because he was certain I had diabetes, instead of Valley Fever, and he scheduled me to come in the following Monday to start learning how to do the injections. I spent the whole weekend agonizing over the fact that I now had diabetes. But when diabetes test results came back after the weekend, and it turned out I tested negative, they canceled the diabetes training. At that point, despite having struggled with some common thyroid symptoms—fatigue, aches, headaches, ups and downs with weight—I still had not had a single thyroid test.

I spent most of my time caring for Spencer, but I did do a little work here and there—at one point, I went to Turkey to do a swimsuit calendar. Then, out of the blue, I had a call about a new pilot for a show called *Sheena*. After *Baywatch*, I wasn't thinking about going back to work on a show, but went to a few meetings with Sony executives, heard them out, and they invited me to shoot the pilot.

I figured, why not? It was just a pilot.

At that point, I was puffy and heavier than I'd like to be on camera, but no one said a word to me. I can't believe it now, looking at pictures of myself back then, especially as Sheena spent the entire pilot episode clad in a skimpy loincloth.

I filmed the pilot—luckily, my mom and Spencer came with

me for the filming. Then I was back to Scottsdale. The health challenges came on stronger than ever. I was having body aches and felt cold all the time—which is pretty shocking in the Arizona heat—and I also noticed I was losing fistfuls of hair. I felt fluish, and still thought maybe I had Valley Fever. As always, I felt exhausted.

Then I found out that *Sheena* was being picked up for a season, and we would be filming in Orlando. My mother agreed to come with Spencer and me for the entire production, and I felt like, with her helping me out, I would be able to make it through.

At this point, my marriage was also beginning to show some cracks, and it was good to leave Scottsdale behind for a while.

I arrived during the summer of 2000, and my first day on the set, I realized I would be earning every dime. It was incredibly hot and humid, and most of the filming was outdoors at MGM studios in Orlando. Every day it was nearly 100 degrees with high humidity. The weather was simply awful and my makeup was running down my face before I even left the chair. I spent a great deal of time on the set worrying about the crew, asking for extra tents and coolers to help them stay cool.

I don't think I'd realized the gravity and workload of being the "star" of a show. They rolled out $30 million to do the show, and it was on me. I was in every scene.

At the same time, it was the most fun I ever had on a production. I became very close to the crew—we were all going through this together. The guys on the camera, the grips on production—they were out there all day, hour after hour, without even a trailer, and we became close. The pressure was intense, and the work was hard, but it was wonderful.

We wrapped the season, and then that fall, I was off to New

York City to do promos. I remember one night, I'd done every show, every radio program, every interview you could imagine, and I was utterly exhausted . . . totally wiped out. I got back to my hotel room at the Peninsula, cleaned off the makeup, and just cried my heart out.

Despite having put heart and soul into *Sheena*, the unreal feeling set in again. This life wasn't really me. I felt like a fake.

"Tonight, let's welcome Gena Fake Nolin. So, Gena, tell us about how awful you feel tonight. And about your sweaty adventures in the jungle. And don't forget to tell us how brain fogged and depressed you feel. Oh, and those extra pounds you're toting around, tell us about it!"

I let it all go, I cried, I was exhausted and felt so alone! I don't think I'd ever really let myself truly feel everything that was going on, the tremendous pressure I felt of trying to make a success starring in my own series.

The heck with it all. I was tired, I hadn't seen my son in a week, and I was realizing, you can't play a lead in a series and be a present, involved mother. Not that actresses don't want to be, but it's just not possible.

But I really couldn't tell anyone how I felt. I had a lot of people working for me on the show, and I felt I needed to be strong for them, and prove to everyone—including myself—that I could do this. Personally, I felt I was living a lie. Behind the walls, my marriage was almost over, and I felt sick, exhausted, and achy. At twenty-nine, all I wanted to do was walk away.

But I didn't. We ultimately filmed twenty-six episodes, and then I found out that *Sheena* was canceled.

Honestly, I was so relieved when it wasn't renewed. But at the same time, it was bittersweet—a time for me to grow up. I had to

cope with the disappointment of having a show canceled and feeling like I let my crew and Sony down, and I worried about how
the crew would feed their families.

Right after *Sheena* was canceled, I was asked by Hugh Hefner
to be in a celebrity pictorial in the 2001 December issue of *Playboy*. I gave it a great deal of thought and looked at some of the
work done by other women in *Playboy*—Marilyn Monroe, Cindy
Crawford, Elle McPherson, Rachel Hunter, Raquel Welch, and so
on. And I said, "Let's do it!"

I had turned them down five times already, but this time was
different. My marriage had ended, I was just turning thirty, it was
now or never! So I whipped myself into shape from the weight
I'd gained on *Sheena*, and made sure I looked good. I made sure
they did everything on my terms, so I had full approval of all photos and the layout. And I arranged for my mother to be with me
throughout it all, standing camera left, making sure it was classy.

We shot a beautiful, sophisticated layout at Bernie Taupin's
ranch in Santa Barbara. Bernie, a friend of Hef's, and Elton John's
longtime songwriting collaborator, wrote the lyrics to most of
Elton's most famous songs. Bernie was the perfect host, telling
us stories from back in the day at amazing restaurants every night
after we shot. Because of *Playboy*, I'm now a piece of history and
proud to be in the company of those amazing women.

I went back to Scottsdale with Spencer, and there, I had to
face the end of my marriage.

Separating from Greg wasn't really a surprise to anyone. Greg
was a good guy, but looking back, I realize that when I met Greg, I
had a lot of healing to do from my childhood. I felt abandoned by
my father, and Greg—older, confident, protective—filled a father
figure role for me at a time when I was young and naive.

And while Greg was the one who pushed me so that I got *The Price Is Right* and *Baywatch*, some of my friends and family feel like he pushed me too hard and never let me relax. My mother has also said that she understands why Greg and I ultimately didn't work as a couple: "Gena didn't really want or plan to get into the entertainment business, but Greg was always there, coming up with new auditions, and cheering her on. She would say, 'I'm tired, I'm ready to drop,' and he would keep pushing her. He's a wonderful businessman and manager, and if wasn't for Greg, she wouldn't have done any of it, but he's a type A personality, and Gena isn't."

Greg also was sometimes dismissive of my health complaints: "Being Canadian, we have this sort of philosophy—if you're not dead, keep moving and don't complain. So I admit, I didn't believe it was something serious. In Arizona, people get Valley Fever, and I figured it might be that. I also wondered if it was depression. I didn't give it much thought at the beginning—because Gena could always do twice as much as everyone else. I figured she was tired or depressed, and she'd get over it, like a cold."

All I knew was that we came to a point when both of us looked at each other and knew it was done, over. I was just turning thirty, and it was time to put my life back together.

Even through Greg and I split, we continued to get along as parents of Spencer, and so, even though I was now a single mother, Greg was involved and took Spencer regularly. I had some free time to explore my new single life.

I didn't think I would ever get married again, but in my entire adult life I had never been single. At thirty, it was time to do what I should have done as a teenager—find out what I was really looking for in a man. By that time, I had great friends, a wonderful tribe of women in Scottsdale who were protective of me. They would set me up on blind dates. Sometimes the guys were intimidated by me, but I was always intimidated by the guys! They had no idea. Being a handsome guy didn't make a difference to me. Looks were low on my list. I discovered that I wanted someone fun, confident, and kind. Meanwhile, I was doubting myself, wondering what he was going to think of a puffy, overweight girl. I used to think, "If they only knew how nervous I am!"

But it didn't stop me from some interesting dates. During a visit to Monaco to present at the World Music Awards, the charming Prince Albert was briefly interested in me, and back in L.A., I had a lovely date with quarterback Tom Brady. Both fellows were true gentlemen.

On the work front, I was being offered every reality show known to man. They wanted me to be in celebrity circuses, go to castaway islands, dance, lose weight, and eat bugs—all of it. When *Fear Factor* called, I thought, "What the heck, I'm going to do it." I was still not back in *Baywatch* shape, but since I wouldn't have to be in a swimsuit, it seemed like it might be an interesting opportunity. So I went on the show and made it through day one, beating out actress Natasha Henstridge. I was thinking, "Great, I'm doing this!"

I was so excited that I had made it through the first day, and when I got to my trailer, they had my wardrobe for the next day laid out. Yes . . . you guessed it. A swimsuit!

We were going to have to swim into an eight-foot tank filled with thousands of snakes—every kind of big snake you can imagine. We had to dive in, grab hockey pucks from the bottom of the tank, and put them in a bucket.

"Oooh, snakes!" you're probably thinking! And yes, the snakes were pretty creepy, but I wasn't as upset about them as I was about appearing in the swimsuit! I was 165 pounds, and it had been a long time since I had appeared publicly in a swimsuit. My face was puffy, my eyelids were puffy, and when I walked out onto the set, I could hear some people actually gasp when they saw me.

It turned out that I wasn't able to get all the pucks during the snakes-in-the-tank challenge, so I got booted. I could have stayed had I eaten a four-inch-long hissing cockroach, but Mom was there in the background, with Spencer, yelling, "Don't do it." There are times when it makes great sense to listen to your mother! I made $10,000 for charity and I left.

After that episode aired, it took no time before radio DJ Howard Stern decided to make me the topic of one of his famous rants. I'd been on Stern's show many times when I was doing *Baywatch*, and we had always had a great time. I thought we had a good relationship.

But he was saying on his show, "Gena Lee Nolin is FAT now." And "So much for the *Baywatch* babe!"

It rocked my confidence, having to be the subject of Stern's ridicule.

Not long after that, I was asked to do *Celebrity Fit Club* for VH1, which had had a couple of successful seasons prior to their asking. I thought I'd do it. They'd heard that I'd gained some weight, and I was willing to do it to get some weight off, and maybe get some buzz.

I signed on for a nice hotel room, lots of working out, and weight loss advice. When I showed up on set, what I ended up with was a cot in an army barrack and an outhouse. They'd changed the format so that this was going to be a "boot camp" but forgot to mention it in the contract! They took my phone, my clothes, everything. They gave me all these skimpy things to wear, to make sure I felt and looked like a total blob. I filmed one episode and contacted my agent. When I explained how much they'd breached the contract, he agreed that I should just leave.

So, adios, *Celebrity Fit Club*. I would have to get fit on my own. How, I didn't know. I was still exhausted, and it seemed that every calorie I ate went straight to my thighs.

Not long after, I was asked to take part in a *Baywatch* reunion movie, filming in Hawaii. After the Howard Stern fiasco, I had a lot of reservations about doing the movie, and the anxiety about being in front of a camera was daunting. But Hassel and the producers really wanted me to do this, and so I finally decided to commit.

I remember being on the set and telling my friend Becky, who was working on the set as a stand-in, that I felt so much bigger than the other actresses.

Becky, however, saw it differently: "Gena was so worried on that set. And I've been around this business for years. Gena looked the best of all the women! She was healthy, and looked normal, not like a bag of bones!"

We were shooting for a month. When we finished, I felt a real sense of accomplishment. I'd done it. Though I wasn't confident going into that film, with the help of friends and a dose of self-confidence, I was able to stand tall.

As they say, it's always darkest before the dawn, and that beautiful sun was about to change my life.

I had a friend, whose husband was a retired hockey player, and she was always setting me up on dates. They'd been fun, but nothing serious. One day she called and said, "Listen Gena, this is it. You have to meet this guy!"

It turned out that through her husband, she knew about this Canadian guy, Cale Hulse, who had just been traded to the Arizona Coyotes hockey team.

I wasn't keen on dating athletes, but she proceeded to give me a laundry list of his amazing qualities: he worked with special needs kids, he mentored mentally challenged people. She probably told me he cured cancer and parted the seas!

"And Gena, he's so tall, even you could wear heels, and he'll still be taller than you."

Hmmm . . . he sounded way too good to be true. So that means he probably was. I was still feeling cynical.

I walked around for a few days with his number, and then finally one day I decided to call him.

"If you really want to meet me, meet me in twenty minutes at Starbucks."

It was a challenge. I was not looking for love, so I put him on the spot. And I didn't make an effort. I went out to Starbucks in a T-shirt, my hair a bit stringy, and I didn't have on an ounce of makeup.

"Screw it," I thought. "If this guy thinks he's going to get the glammed-up *Baywatch* girl, let's see what he thinks of the REAL me! AND, let's see if I even like him anyway!"

I walked into Starbucks and there was this six-foot-three blond Adonis—how else can I describe him? And my first thought was, "Oh my gosh, what was I thinking? Why didn't I wear any makeup?!"

We sat there at Starbucks and talked for three hours straight. Cale was my type of guy, and I knew it from the start. He was down to earth, insightful, compassionate, very sweet—not at all a typical athlete. Clearly, we were hitting it off.

My friend Janell remembers how I called her right after the date: "I could tell from Gena's voice that he was something special. And it was so Gena, to show up for a date wearing no makeup and a T-shirt, her hair in a ponytail, and to end up with the man of her dreams!"

Cale tells the story from his perspective:

I met Gena on my first and only blind date in my life. I had just come to the Phoenix area to play for the Coyotes, after playing in Nashville. A friend of a friend thought that I should meet Gena. We agreed to meet for coffee, but hadn't set a date. She called me at the last minute, and asked me if I wanted to meet at Starbucks in fifteen minutes. I said why not. The interesting thing is, I am probably one of the only guys out there who really didn't know who she was. And honestly, since it was my first blind date, I didn't get my hopes up.

But I knew from the moment she walked in the door. I was hoping to meet a down-to-earth, real person, and there she was. Hours went by, and it felt like five minutes. I was so impressed with Gena, with her warmth, personality, and her natural beauty. And it was clear that I didn't care about Hollywood, and she didn't care about hockey, but we were definitely interested in each other that day over coffee. I asked her out to dinner for the next evening, and we have been together ever since.

Cale and I were getting serious, but I waited many months before introducing him to Spencer. Finally, I told Spencer that a friend of mine I have coffee with was going to come for dinner. Spencer was six, and in typical kid fashion, he said, "OK, whatever." He didn't realize how important this dinner was.

Cale actually made dinner—he's quite the cook—and Cale, Spencer, and I were sitting there around the table when Spence announced, "Ewww . . . this tastes like dog food!"

I was thinking, OK, that's it. Cale's definitely going to run for the hills!

Cale leaned over to Spencer and said, "Hey, buddy, how do you know what dog food tastes like?"

Spencer looked up at him, wide-eyed, and then laughed.

From that point on, they had a love affair . . . they'd play in the pool and hang out together. I think they fell in love before Cale and I did. Cale and Spence were effortless together; this was how it was supposed to go. Cale was also helping Spencer cope with his recent diagnosis of ADD, teaching Spence to center himself, be calm, and focus.

My standards were high, and I knew that any relationship had to be right or nothing. And Cale was right. I really loved how humble he was. He was so unassuming about his achievements and his athletic prowess. He was a soft-spoken, gentle giant. He worked hard, and when he had to show his stuff, he always delivered at every training camp. He also had no idea how handsome he was. Tall, gorgeous, an amazing build, and the guy had no clue. He was also generous, and would give you the proverbial shirt off his back.

Most of all, I loved his character, what he stood for, what he believed in.

In March 2004, Cale and I had been dating for six months, and things were going so well, frankly, it was perfect! And when things are perfect, well, you know how it goes. Don't they say there's always calm before a storm?

I had a phone call from Jerry, my PR guy, and it was not good news. A videotape had been leaked, and I was in it. "*Baywatch Babe Sex Tape*" was about to hit the tabloid headlines.

Greg and I had filmed it when we were newlyweds, just goofing around with a new video camera. I had forgotten about it. But it seemed that someone in Greg's family who needed the money had found the tape and decided to cash in by selling it to the tabloids.

The first thing I thought of was my son. How could I protect him from this? And the next thing I thought about was Cale. I felt humiliated, and I was certain that the second he caught wind of this—he was on the road playing an away game—he would understandably dump me.

I called Cale, and through tears, I told him what had happened. Cale said he would call me right back, and I was thinking, "This is it. When he calls back, he's going to dump me."

He called me back and said, "You know what . . . you were a married woman. I'm madly in love with you and this is in no way going to shake our relationship. We'll get through this together."

At that moment, I just fell to my knees, dropped the phone, and started crying.

I realized that I finally had a man who loved me unconditionally—who accepted me exactly as I was. He understood the situation, and that was it. He would stand by me.

Cale says he still remembers that call like it was yesterday.

I was in a hotel for an away game. Gena called, and I could tell from her voice that something was wrong—she could barely talk through her tears. It broke my heart to hear how sad and afraid she was. But my immediate reaction was protectiveness. I had come to realize how rare and special our relationship was, and how incredible Gena was. So I knew it was just a bump in the road . . . something we would get through, and past, together.

So we rode out the storm of the tape, and within a year, Cale and I were engaged, and three months after we got engaged, I proudly walked down the aisle and married the love of my life.

At our wedding, everyone knew the story of our first meeting at a Starbucks. Many of the single ladies were repeating what ended up being the funniest line of the night: "By the way, the next time I'm at Starbucks, I want a nonfat Cale Hulse!"

I discovered that my marriage to Cale was the first healthy relationship with a man that I'd ever had. And I loved that. We both came to the marriage deciding to give 100 percent. That way, we couldn't go wrong.

Athletes can have their downsides, but with Cale, he brought a team player mentality that was so great. He always has seen himself as part of a team, not a star player, and that earns him the respect of his fellow players. I think it's because of his willingness to be unselfish, to give, to do whatever it takes to help the team win.

Cale has always been a team player! Marriage was a segue for him, from sports to marriage and family life. His new family became his new team.

An important part of our family was Caia, Cale's daughter. She increasingly spent more time with us in Scottsdale, and on our travels. I got to know Caia and discovered what a wonderful young lady she was, and we grew to love each other. I felt like her second mother, just like Cale truly became a second father to Spencer.

3

It's Complicated

The greater the difficulty, the more the glory in surmounting it.
—EPICURUS

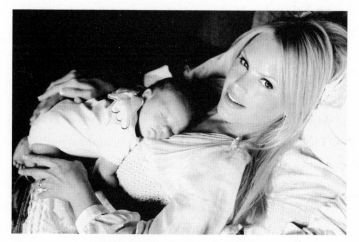

With three-week-old Stella Monroe

After Cale and I got married, we decided to try to have a baby. We were excited, and since I thought of myself as a "fertile Myrtle"— I got pregnant with Spencer on the first try—I was thrilled when I again got pregnant right away. We went in for an ultrasound at around nine weeks. The woman performing the ultrasound and the other medical assistant were looking back and forth at each other, and they didn't say anything. Cale and I were suspicious, but the doctor stuck his head in, and said, "Just go home and enjoy being pregnant."

Within two days, I started miscarrying, and it was horrible, painful, emotionally draining . . . an awful thing to experience. I really believe that they saw this was going to happen, or knew that pregnancy probably wasn't viable, but they didn't tell me.

I felt like a fool and a failure, and incomplete. Cale was upset and supportive. I was worried that I might never be able to have a baby with Cale.

We waited about five months before we started trying again, and I quickly got pregnant again.

This time, the pregnancy continued.

During this time, Cale was playing hockey in Columbus, and we had a rental condo there, where I was staying. I became obsessed with the Melting Pot restaurant, where they serve fondue dishes. There was one right across the street, and I was there three nights a week. The waiters knew me . . . and believe me, they did not like me! I would waddle over there with or without Cale, and order chocolate fondue. One time I was there on my own, and I was sure they'd short-changed me on my chocolate, and I complained loudly.

The waiter said "Listen, ma'am, it's premeasured."

"I swear I had more chocolate last week!" I yelled.

Clearly, I was obsessed with chocolate . . . and a little bit hormonal. (You think?!)

I had started out this pregnancy heavier, and gained even more—some of it clearly thanks to chocolate fondue!—but except for the occasional run-in with the Melting Pot waiters, it was a happy pregnancy. Cale was dedicated, devoted, and, surprisingly to me, he found me sexy. I naturally felt self-conscious about getting big, and I carried very wide, but Cale loved me exactly the way I was. It means all the difference in the world when you have that nurturing and support. He would tell me I looked beautiful. As a result, my libido was crazy while carrying Hudson—it had never been stronger. Cale was happy—after he'd been traveling for road games, we'd come back together, and it would be a week of cheese fondue, chocolate fondue, and sex. I had a pair of crazy-hot designer maternity jeans—a major splurge that I recommend for all pregnant women—that I just about lived in. I was as big as a barrel, I had the Melting Pot across the street, and life was good! We were very much in love, and very happy.

Around the time I was due to give birth, Cale was playing for the Calgary Flames, and we had been apart for six weeks. I couldn't fly at the end of the pregnancy, and I didn't know if he'd be back for the birth. But he arranged with his coach to let him leave the team early, and surprised me by arriving home two days before delivery was induced. He wasn't going to miss the birth of his baby!

In the end, I had to have an emergency C-section, but baby Hudson was beautiful and healthy. Cale had tears rolling down his face when he first saw him.

I was happy but exhausted. I had baby Hudson and Spencer, and was keeping it all going mainly on my own. Cale was on the road, playing hockey; I was blessed, though, in that I had some help, where a lot of people don't. I had a nurse a few nights a week so I could get a full night's sleep.

After Hudson was born, my health problems seemed to come roaring back with a vengeance. I now know that it was a flare-up of Hashimoto's disease—this autoimmune disease can calm down during pregnancy, but frequently gets far worse or appears for the first time right after pregnancy. I was exhausted in a way I'd never experienced before. When I saw pictures of myself, it was obvious how puffy and bloated I was.

Despite watching what I ate, and getting more exercise, my weight was fluctuating. I would drag myself to the gym and was eating carefully, and finally, at the point when I had lost almost all the pregnancy weight, my symptoms got worse again, and I started gaining weight again. I was up to 180 pounds, the most I'd ever weighed except when I was pregnant with Spencer. I was exhausted, my joints and muscles were sore and achy, my lymph nodes were swollen. (I have an uncle who has a twenty-year history of lymphoma, and I was so sick, I worried that maybe I had it, too.) The doctors kept running blood tests—never for thyroid, of course—and said they couldn't find anything wrong.

Looking back, it's clear that Hashimoto's disease had gone into full gear after Hudson's birth, but, like many women, I struggled with the symptoms and remained undiagnosed.

Cale and I were invited to Hugh Hefner's famed Midsummer Night's Eve party at the Playboy Mansion. It's one of his biggest annual parties, and everyone has to wear a negligee or pajamas. Not necessarily sexy lingerie—some people wear cozy jammies.

So I got a pretty robe with matching pajamas, nothing too sexy, but not too dowdy, and waltzed into the Playboy Mansion with Cale, thinking I looked pretty cute.

The first person I ran into was Jane's Addiction guitarist Dave Navarro, who had married Carmen Electra, an actress I'd worked with on *Baywatch*.

I smiled and said hi to Dave, and he just looked at me. We had hung out together in the past, but it became clear that he had absolutely no idea who I was.

Even Hef didn't know it was me. "It's Gena!" I had to say to him.

It was awkward beyond belief. I knew I was chubby, but I was in a different place in my life. I was married, happy, with children. And yet I thought I should fit right in at this party.

Cale told me later that there were awful looks, whispers, and comments all night. I was really oblivious, and, frankly, am so glad he didn't tell me at the time.

I realized how fickle it all was. Hollywood was so much about what you look like, what you are doing right this moment. Are you current? Are you aging well? And if you don't look a certain way, you're simply invisible. It's very simple.

Not a single person at that party said, "Hey, Gena, how are you doing?" Instead, the conversation was all superficial.

But it is what it is . . . it's an industry based on who's who, and it's a game. When you're on top, everyone wants you and adores you, but if you come in looking a certain way or you're not on a hit show anymore, you're toast.

More than anything though, the whole Playboy party scene was a real awakening to me, as far as my illness and how it had taken me over. I took a long, hard look at myself in the mirror. I was very puffy, my eyelids were swollen, my weight was up, and I was constantly exhausted. Something was seriously wrong, but I didn't know where I would find the energy to get back into yet another endless round of doctor visits.

Still, despite how I felt, Cale and I wanted to have another baby.

I very much wanted to have a girl, so I got all these books, read up on the Internet, and found different techniques to help increase your odds of conceiving a girl.

I'd read this old wives' tale that said that if the man ejaculates three to four days prior to ovulation, it increases the odds for a girl. We tried it. And I know it's not scientific, but after having two boys, I tried this approach, got pregnant, and an ultrasound later revealed that it was a girl! We decided to call her Stella Monroe.

When I was pregnant with Stella, something strange happened to my body. Instead of my usual weight gain, I was losing weight. I now recognize that what I was going through was a period of hyperthyroidism, an overactive thyroid. I felt anxious, and the weight was falling off. I didn't have much of an appetite.

When I was just six weeks pregnant, I remember sitting with a friend one day, when I realized that I couldn't catch my breath, and I was feeling anxious. Just walking into her house had felt like I had just run a marathon and was dragging myself over the finish line. I realized that I was having some sort of heart palpitations, so I drove myself to the ER, and they admitted me. From that point on, they tried to figure out what was the matter—and that's when they first told me that I was having atrial fibrillation, a fast and erratic heart rhythm. If it became uncontrolled, it could cause a heart attack, stroke, or even death. They sent me home with a prescription beta-blocker in case it happened again, and said if that didn't work, to come back to the ER.

For a while, my heart stayed in control, but I was very anxious—I felt very hyper and nervous. I didn't gain much weight—I was much slimmer during this pregnancy compared to Hudson's and Spencer's. Looking back, it was obviously hyperthyroid.

I had another episode of atrial fibrillation and they hospitalized me for three days, then sent me off to a cardiologist, where I sat in the waiting room with a big group of senior citizens. The stress tests and EKG said everything was fine.

At seven months, I was at the gym, doing a light workout. Cale was with me that day. I was listening to my iPod, walking on the treadmill, and I suddenly realized I couldn't catch my breath. My heart was pounding out of my chest, so I slowed down, and I still couldn't catch my breath. I got off the treadmill, and Cale had me lie down on a mat and put some ice on my neck. My pulse was erratic and fast—close to 200 beats per minute. Cale took me to the ER.

Since I was pregnant and this was my second trip to the ER, they admitted me immediately. I was there for five days while they tried various medications, but nothing was working. Nothing was getting the heart rhythm under control.

At this point, they did a basic thyroid check, which they said was normal. I don't know if they checked antibodies or circulating thyroid levels—I highly doubt it, actually. And I wish they had, because my doctors have subsequently said that spending an entire pregnancy with Hashimoto's antibodies, my thyroid going in and out of hyperthyroidism, was probably the cause of the atrial fibrillation.

Cale and I were terrified. He is usually stoic and handles pressure and stress with great calm. But while I was in the hospital, there were times I caught him looking at me, in that hospital bed, and I could see the fear in his eyes. I was hooked up to every monitor in the joint, and they still couldn't figure it out.

Cale did everything he could to be supportive. I remember him saying, "I'm here, I love you, and we'll get through this. There's nothing we can't get through. We'll get to the bottom of this . . . we'll get you healthy."

A cardiologist came in and said, "We don't usually do this with a pregnant woman, but we're going to have to cardiovert you—you know, with the paddles. It's just a split second."

I immediately thought, "No way." The only other option was to try another medication. They brought in an expert on high-risk pregnancy, and they decided to give me a strong dose of digoxin—a class C drug (a digitalis derivative) they didn't typically use in pregnancy. "We're not sure what it does to the baby, but it's the only other option."

Luckily, the digoxin worked, but I worried what it might do to Stella. I still remember the tears pouring down my face.

My current physician, Dr. Alan Christianson, believes that my atrial fibrillation was very likely related to my undiagnosed and untreated Hashimoto's thyroiditis. "The high hormone levels of pregnancy can impede thyroid function further during pregnancy. When you add in the immunologic changes—a pregnant woman's body has to accommodate the presence of the fetus, which is essentially 'foreign'—a whole autoimmune cascade can manifest, and that can include cardiac symptoms like Gena experienced."

I got through that episode, but those last months were nerve-racking. I never knew if another episode would start up again. Because I'd had a C-section with Hudson, they scheduled me for a C-section to deliver Stella. I know I started to have some a-fib again right before the epidural, but it calmed down enough for me to deliver Stella.

My daughter came out screaming. She's a beautiful, bright little girl, but she is very strong-willed, and very intense. I still wonder if the digoxin had an effect on her. But what choice did I have? If they hadn't treated the a-fib, I could have died, and Stella could have died. I hope and pray that she stays as healthy as she is. She's such a special little girl, and I can't imagine my life without her.

After Stella was born, I was now mother to a houseful of children. We had Spencer, Hudson, and baby Stella, and Caia was with us regularly, usually for weeks at a time.

I struggled to keep up, breast-feeding Stella, getting Spencer off to school, and keeping track of Hudson, who was an incredibly active little boy.

And I felt more and more exhausted.

I had committed to doing a "Body after Baby" photo shoot for *People* magazine after Stella's birth, so, tired as I was, I did everything I could to get in shape for the photo shoot. Looking back at those pictures, I don't know if I was ever in that good shape before or since!

When Stella was seven months old, we were spending the summer in California. We went to Manhattan Beach for a fun family day and were walking up the hill from the beach. I realized I couldn't catch my breath, so I walked a bit more, and then stopped and felt my pulse. It was erratic and racing. I said, "Cale, I'm not going to jump to conclusions," and had him feel my pulse.

Immediately, he said, "I'm getting the car." He rushed me to the emergency room, where they discovered I was in a-fib again. They hooked me up to an IV to bring it back into rhythm. Luckily, that's the last time I've had to deal with atrial fibrillation, and believe me, I'm hoping it never happens again.

After that episode, I decided that I had had it.

I had a consult with a well-known doctor. I still remember him coming in to the examining room, and he told me quite condescendingly that I needed to see a psychiatrist. "You need to stop coming in, there is absolutely nothing wrong with you!"

I was intimidated, so I nodded my head, tears dropping as I left his office. I was afraid to call the office again, because I'd heard the office staff referring to me as "*Baywatch*." If I called, they'd be saying, "Oh, *Baywatch* is calling again . . ."

I saw another doctor who was apparently a fan of mine. He was quick to tell me that he had just been looking at some magazine pictures of me right before coming in to the examining room. Can you say "inappropriate"? I wanted to get up and run right out of the examining room. I didn't, though I should have. But I never went back to him.

I just wanted to find a doctor who would believe me, and would tell me that I was going to be okay.

I've watched girlfriends go through breast cancer, and I was always encouraging them never to leave a stone unturned, never to give up on themselves. I told them that if something doesn't feel right, it's probably because it's not right. But it was harder to apply that good advice to myself, as I went from doctor to doctor, disappointed and afraid.

Finally, one day, I got a call from the latest doctor I'd seen.

I'll never forget the message he left. He said, "Your thyroid levels are a bit high."

I was thrilled. Here, I finally had some sort of answer, some hope!

But the rest of the message went on. "But I'm not going to medicate you, because then you'll have to take it the rest of your life."

He had figured out something was wrong with me, but he wasn't going to treat me?!

When I went in to see him, he brushed me off like it was nothing: "Maybe in a year you should recheck it, and if it's any higher, start medication."

I hung up, immediately called my obstetrician, and asked him to help interpret. According to Dr. "Wait Ten Years," I had a thyroid-stimulating hormone (TSH) value of 7. A normal level runs from around 0.5 to 4.5. The OB said that it was indeed high enough to treat.

He was willing to treat me, and he started me on a drug called Synthroid.

From pictures of myself at the time, it is clear how hypothyroid I was. My neck was enlarged, my face bloated, and my eyelids so puffy you could barely see my eyes. I was battling twenty extra pounds that I'd gained in less than two months.

It didn't make sense. I was being treated, but I was still so sick; I can't even explain how terrible I felt. Every day it was, "Surprise! Here's a new symptom!" First it was puffy eyes, then puffy face, more exhaustion, hair loss, and those oh-so-lovely mood swings. I was bloated. My joints ached. I was on the couch, shivering, buried under covers and blankets; I was freezing; my throat was burning and enlarged; I felt dizzy; and I could barely stand. The strangest thing was that I had also developed a fear and anxiety about social interactions. It was so not like me. I'm a good actress . . . I'm outgoing. I can go into a room and talk, chat, and connect very easily. And here I was, barely able to get out of bed, unable to put together a sentence, and dreading being around people.

Cale was especially worried about me.

I knew she'd been struggling, but when she was finally diagnosed, I think the first reaction I felt was fear—the fear of not knowing much about what she had, how serious it was, whether it was treatable, and would there be side effects? I also worried about her emotionally, because I know how seriously she takes being mother to our children. It was breaking her heart that she wasn't able to muster the energy to give our little ones her full-time attention. You take things for granted healthwise until someone you care about more than anything is diagnosed with a disease.

A few months later, the obstetrician recommended that I see an endocrinologist—a thyroid specialist.

Again, I was thrilled. Finally, an expert who would finally get to the bottom of my symptoms!

At the consultation with the endocrinologist, she felt my gland, had me do a "thyroid neck check" swallow test, and also did an ultrasound scan because she felt something on my thyroid. Lo and behold, the scan showed that I had a pretty good size solid nodule in my thyroid.

The next step was a fine-needle aspiration biopsy. My husband went with me, and while the doctor had this needle going into my throat, I was worrying that I might have cancer. I'd gone from "everything is fine," to "high TSH," to "suspicious nodule," and it felt overwhelming.

During the biopsy, they confirmed that I had Hashimoto's thyroiditis and it had atrophied the entire right side of my thyroid gland. The autoimmune disease had almost completely shut down my thyroid.

I then had to wait until the day before Thanksgiving of 2009, when I finally got the call. I was in Boston doing an appearance, I felt run-down and fluish, and my thyroid was sore from the biopsy. I was on pins and needles waiting for the results. In the business office on the hotel computer, I searched for information about thyroid nodules: "95 percent are benign," "thyroid cancer treatments," "radioactive iodine," and so on. It was hard to console me, though, because no one knew what was going on with me.

The doctor's assistant called and was really sweet. "Your results are coming through the fax right now." The doctor got on the phone, and said, "It's benign!" I was thrilled. That was a year I definitely had something to give thanks for.

But even with my nodule in the clear, my symptoms continued. I went back to the endocrinologist and told her how weak and exhausted I felt.

The doctor tried to muster some sympathy, but she didn't really have any suggestions. I left that appointment so weak and out of it that I couldn't even drive home. I called Cale, and his parents were in town. He and his dad came to pick me up. I'm sure they thought I was a hypochondriac, but I couldn't figure out any other way to get home.

After going through multiple doctors, tests, and scans—at one point, one of the doctors even did an MRI of my brain—I was being written off again.

My current doctor, Alan Christianson, says, "It feels like having the flu all the time." It's no surprise I felt so sick. But no one had told me this.

I was lost. I knew that no one believed me, and apparently, there wasn't anything dire, like a cancerous tumor, but I needed to find a way back.

ADVOCACY

I mustered what energy I did have and started reading. I turned to the computer and read everything I could find on Hashimoto's disease and hypothyroidism. I read websites, articles, medical journals. I bought books. I didn't always understand everything, but I understood enough to recognize that I'd had thyroid symptoms for almost twenty years, and no one had ever checked my thyroid until after Stella was born.

That's also when I found Mary Shomon. I would type in "thyroid," and up would come Mary, her articles, blogs, and books. And everything I read would hit home. Mary got me.

I found my way to Mary's Thyroid Support page on Facebook, and I started reading what other thyroid patients were saying. I saw the different conversations, and people chiming in, and it was as if I had written every post.

I finally knew I was home.

I started posting, and people shared their ideas and experiences with me.

Armed with new information, I went to my doctor and demanded every test he had. Everything came back "normal," and at that point, I knew I had nothing left to lose, and so I told him I had to change to a new medication, a natural desiccated thyroid drug called Armour Thyroid. The doctor agreed, and on New Year's Day of 2010, I started my new thyroid medication. Within a few days, it was, well, wow! I was finally starting to come back to life.

For me, switching to the natural thyroid medication proved to be a turning point, and slowly, I felt my energy returning, the brain fog lifting, and my health starting to improve.

I wanted to share my experiences with others, but I was discovering that few people—even friends and family—truly understood the toll that thyroid disease had taken and was still taking on my life.

Actually, it started to seem like *no one* even wanted to talk about it, except for me! I think it was a combination of being really excited that I was finally starting to feel better, and also determined that others should not have to go through what I went through. I had been misdiagnosed and poorly treated for so long, but now I had some answers. So I wanted to talk about thyroid disease all the time, with everyone. I wanted to shout from the rooftops, "Get your thyroid tested!" I know, it was a bit over the top. There I was, going on about thyroid this, and thyroid that. It got to the point when sometimes, on girls' night out, my friends were looking at me and saying, "Ummm, Gena, can we *please NOT* talk about your thyroid tonight?" Even my husband, who has been so patient, would sometimes say, "I love you, but I just can't listen to another thyroid story."

As I learned how to have more control over my thyroid condition, through trial and error, I began to explore what sort of thyroid awareness activities were taking place. There I was, eager to share my thyroid story, and tell everyone I know to find good doctors, get their thyroids tested, and get treated. I was looking around and talking to many of the people I know in the entertainment business, and I was hearing about all these people who have thyroid conditions. *So why wasn't anyone talking about it in public?*

Where were the national thyroid awareness ribbons and bracelets? Where were the 5K runs and walks and bicycle rides for thyroid disease? Where were the fund-raising events? Why wasn't it regularly discussed on talk shows, the local news health segments, and in women's magazines?

Every time I saw a story about the causes of infertility, or postpartum depression, or weight gain, all I could think was, why wasn't anyone mentioning thyroid?

I began to realize that this disease that had plagued me for two decades was one that has an unfortunate and mysterious stigma. Thyroid disease was a problem most people just don't want to talk about . . . and *especially* not celebrities.

I got it. This was not a pretty disease; at its worst, it's not a sexy disease. When we think about Hashimoto's and hypothyroidism, we think of depression, weight struggles, thinning hair, fatigue, and aches and pains. There's nothing glamorous about being depressed and tired all the time. There's nothing glamorous about hair that looks and feels like straw. And forget about struggling to stay slim. When you think about it, thyroid disease is a total nightmare for someone in the entertainment business. I know, because I lived it. So it's no wonder that most celebrity thyroid patients are actively trying to hide it, instead of going public.

There was no question that I was sick of being sick. But I was also incredibly relieved. I finally had the answer as to why I'd felt this way for twenty years. Finally, I knew I wasn't crazy, I *wasn't* a hypochondriac . . . I didn't have to go this alone.

But as I read the posts from other women, my heart was breaking. I realized that my own thyroid nightmare—the struggle to get diagnosed, to find doctors, to find the right treatment, and to cope with the ups and downs and visible signs of the chronic disease—was the same nightmare that millions of other women were experiencing every day.

Those women were still living through what I'd experienced for twenty years. They deserved that same relief, that same understanding that they are not alone in this struggle.

I decided that I wanted to create a community, a place where I could blog, share some of the things I'd learned, and share my thyroid journey with others who were on that same crazy trip.

That's when the name *Thyroid Sexy* came to me, and soon, my Thyroid Sexy page on Facebook was born, and it took off. I called it Thyroid Sexy because it was the most unsexy I had ever felt, and I knew I needed inspiration, and thought I might inspire others.

There were so many answers, and so much information, but you had to know what was wrong in the first place. And then you had to be willing to dive in, develop some backbone when dealing with doctors, stand up for yourself. I wanted to have a place to talk, to feel comfortable. I wanted to pay it forward. I'm so touched when I see that someone has gotten the support, information, or help they need.

And at that point I decided that I had to do even more. There was a huge vacuum in the area of thyroid awareness—a space for a celebrity to help create awareness of thyroid disease among people who may not know much, or even realize they had a thyroid condition. I knew it was my mission to use whatever celebrity I had to help raise thyroid awareness, and encourage others to be empowered and informed.

I emailed Mary Shomon. We got on the phone a few days later, and, well, you know what happened next . . . this book!

Now I have a new purpose and direction. And my family and friends—even my doctor—have been so supportive of my role as an advocate, and are excited about this new direction in my life.

Cale, my husband, partner, and love of my life, is convinced that this book, and my other awareness activities, are a positive step.

People see Gena, and beyond her obvious beauty, talent, and business savvy, most people don't know that Gena has such a big heart, and how caring and loving she is. She is one of the most compassionate people I've ever met, whether with me, the children, and our family. So many women suffer from thyroid disease, and are undiagnosed and misdiagnosed, like Gena was, so awareness is crucial. Once people are more aware, the understanding will come, and I think that will be a key part of the healing process for Gena. Gena is putting emphasis on the things that truly matter most in our lives.

My mom, Patricia, has also been a big support. "I wasn't surprised that Gena is moving into the role of an advocate. She's been in this role of star this, body that, beautiful this and that, but I really believe it was all part of a much deeper life journey. There's a lot more to Gena than looking good in a swimsuit. And now that she's turned forty, she's headed in a new direction. She's helping make people more aware, and along the way, smile and laugh."

Greg has been supportive as well.

I was and remain proud of Gena's efforts in thyroid advocacy. She has even told me that she's wondered if the real purpose of her earlier celebrity was to give her a platform to help others. She really feels a social responsibility to get the message out, to share the frustrations she experienced, to help others take a harder look.

Athletes and celebrities get people doing colonoscopies, prostate exams, mammograms, and such, and they can be real conduits to doing something important for your health. Gena is playing that role for thyroid patients. If one person gets the right treatment and health improvement, Gena has made an impact and changed someone's life for the better.

I've got a new role, perhaps the real role of a lifetime! I am a thyroid patient advocate.

And now it's time for me to start doing some nitty-gritty advocacy. Let's get started!

Part 2

THE NITTY-GRITTY

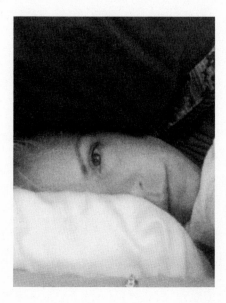

4

Thyroid 101

There are two sides to every question.

—PROTAGORAS

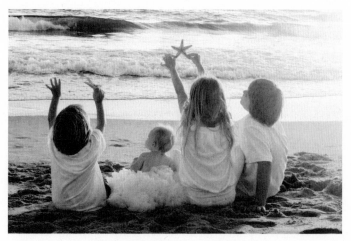

Hudson, Stella, Caia, and Spencer

I can't say that I gave a whole lot of thought to the issue of hormones before my thyroid problem was diagnosed. But nowadays, you can't shut me up when I get started talking about the endocrine system and hormones and how they affect your mind, body, and well-being. I'm a living example of how they can turn your life upside down.

If you, like me, didn't go to med school—heck, I never even played a doctor on TV!—the whole thing is probably totally confusing, so let's take a look at some of the need-to-know basics about the thyroid.

ENDOCRINE 101 CRASH COURSE

Let's start with the endocrine system. It is made up of organs and glands that primarily serve to release hormones. The major endocrine organs and glands in women, their location, and some of the key hormones they release, include:

- Pineal gland, located in the brain, releases melatonin.
- Pituitary gland, located in the brain, releases thyroid-stimulating hormone (TSH), growth hormone (GH), endorphins, follicle-stimulating hormone (FSH), luteinizing hormone (LH), and others.
- Thyroid gland, located in the neck, releases primarily thyroxine (T4) and triiodothyronine (T3).
- Parathyroid glands, located next to the thyroid in the neck, release parathyroid hormone (PTH).
- Thymus, located in the chest, releases thymosins, hormones that help immune system cells function.
- Adrenal glands, located over the kidneys, release cortisol, adrenaline (epinephrine), noradrenaline (norepinephrine), dopamine, testosterone, and others.
- Pancreas, located in the abdominal area, releases insulin, glucagon, and other hormones.
- Ovaries, located in the pelvic region, release reproductive hormones, including estrogens, progesterone, testosterone, dehydroepiandrosterone (DHEA), and others.
- The hypothalamus, located in the brain, functions as both

part of the endocrine system and the nervous system, and acts as a link between them. The hypothalamus coordinates the endocrine system overall, releasing hormones to help control the other glands' activities and acting to coordinate the various glands and hormonal cycles. Another key function of the hypothalamus is triggering the starting point for the female menstrual cycle.

UNDERSTANDING YOUR THYROID

Let's move on to the thyroid. I have to tell you, I didn't know a thing about the thyroid, even after I was diagnosed. It was only after I'd been diagnosed for a while and was getting treated but still struggling that I hit the computer and started Googling, then reading. And holy cow, did I have my eyes opened wide. That was really the beginning of a whole new life for me, learning about thyroid disease and understanding what was going on in my body.

I don't want you to wait as long as I did to get the basics. So here goes.

First, the thyroid is a small gland located in your neck near the windpipe. It's shaped like a butterfly—that's why you'll see butterflies often used as a symbol for the thyroid, and I have one in the Thyroid Sexy community logo as well.

This little butterfly-shaped gland's job is to produce several hormones, but there are two biggies: triiodothyronine (don't even try to pronounce it, just call it T3) and thyroxine (known as T4). These hormones help oxygen get into your cells and are essential to your body's ability to produce energy. Let's repeat that. Oxygen and energy. Pretty important, right? The thyroid is the master gland of your metabolism!

The thyroid absorbs iodine from our food, salt, and supplements, and combined with an amino acid, tyrosine, it makes mostly T4 hormone, and some T3 hormone. T4 is the storage hormone, and T3 is the active hormone that goes into the cells. So the rest of the T3 needed by the body is supposed to be formed as the body converts T4 into T3. Once T3 reaches your cells, it helps convert oxygen and calories into energy to serve as your body's fuel.

How does the thyroid know how much T4 and T3 to produce? It's all part of a feedback loop. The hypothalamus, a part of the brain, releases something called thyrotropin-releasing hormone (TRH). The release of TRH tells your pituitary gland to in turn produce thyroid-stimulating hormone (TSH). The TSH that circulates in your bloodstream is the messenger that is supposed to tell your thyroid to make the thyroid hormones T4 and T3 and send them into your bloodstream. When the pituitary senses that you have enough thyroid hormone circulating, the pituitary makes less TSH. The reduction in TSH signals to the thyroid that it can slow down thyroid hormone production. When the pituitary senses that there is not enough thyroid hormone circulating, TSH goes up again.

It's a smoothly functioning system when it works properly. But when the thyroid gland doesn't work properly, or something gets in the way of this whole process, look out!

In the United States, the most common cause of a thyroid problem is Hashimoto's disease, the autoimmune condition that causes the body to produce antibodies that attack, chip away at, and, if untreated, eventually destroy the thyroid. This results in hypothyroidism, the most common thyroid condition in the United States. Hypothyroidism means your thyroid gland is not producing enough—or any—thyroid hormone. Some people end up hypothyroid because they have their thyroid surgically removed—after cancer or for nodules. And sometimes, the thyroid slows or shuts down after radioactive iodine treatment for an overactive thyroid.

Besides hypothyroidism, there are several other things that can go wrong with the thyroid, including:

- Hyperthyroidism—when the thyroid is overactive and is producing too much thyroid hormone
- Goiter—when the thyroid becomes enlarged, due to hypothyroidism or hyperthyroidism
- Nodules—when lumps, usually benign, grow in the thyroid, sometimes causing it to become hypo- or hyperthyroid
- Thyroid cancer—when lumps or nodules in the thyroid are malignant
- Postpartum thyroiditis—when the thyroid is temporarily inflamed, in addition to hypo- or hyperthyroidism triggered after pregnancy

Both Mary and I have Hashimoto's thyroiditis and the resulting hypothyroidism. I also have thyroid nodules, which are common in Hashimoto's patients.

I didn't realize it at first, but I had several key risk factors for a thyroid problem, including a family history of thyroid problems, plus I grew up in the Midwest, where the soil is low in iodine, and thyroid problems are more prevalent there.

Other risk factors to keep in mind:

- You or someone in your family has a history of autoimmune disease (e.g., rheumatoid arthritis, psoriasis, vitiligo, multiple sclerosis, lupus, or other conditions).
- You are or were a smoker.
- You have allergies or a sensitivity to gluten, or have been diagnosed with celiac disease.
- You've been exposed to radiation—from living near or downwind from a nuclear plant, or have had radioactive medical treatments (e.g., treatment for Hodgkin's disease, nasal radium therapy, radiation to tonsils and neck area), or have had too many dental or neck X-rays (without a thyroid collar), or you were nearby or downwind of the Chernobyl nuclear disaster in 1986.
- You've been treated with lithium (for bipolar disorder, or amiodarone (for heart rhythm problems).
- You have been taking supplements that include iodine, kelp, bladder wrack, and/or bugleweed.
- You've been exposed to excessive amounts of environmental estrogens, chemicals, and toxins (e.g., perchlorate, fluoride, bisphenol-A) via your water, food, or your job.
- You drink fluoridated water and use external fluoride (fluoridated toothpaste, fluoride treatments).
- You eat a lot of soy products, especially processed soy or soy-based supplements.
- You eat or juice a lot of raw "goitrogenic" veggies, such as Brussels sprouts, rutabaga, turnips, kohlrabi, radishes, cauliflower, cabbage, and kale.
- You are over sixty.
- You are female.
- You are in a period of hormonal change—like peri-

menopause (40+), menopause (50+), pregnancy, or post-partum.
• You have had serious trauma to the neck, such as whiplash from a car accident or a broken neck.

THYROID TESTING

One test you can do yourself, at home, is a thyroid neck check. This simple self-test can potentially detect some thyroid abnormalities. To do the thyroid neck check, hold a mirror so that you can see your thyroid area—just below the Adam's apple and above the collarbone. Tip your head back, while keeping this view of your neck and thyroid area visible in your mirror. Take a drink of water and swallow. As you swallow, look at your neck. Watch carefully for any bulges, enlargement, protrusions, or unusual appearances in this area. Repeat this process several times. If you see anything that appears unusual, see your doctor right away. You may have a goiter (an enlarged thyroid) or a thyroid nodule, and your thyroid should be evaluated. (Be sure you don't get your Adam's apple confused with your thyroid gland. The Adam's apple is right at the front of your neck; the thyroid is farther down, closer to your collarbone.) Remember that this is not a conclusive test. You can still have a thyroid problem even if nothing is visible.

You can also measure your basal temperature. A chronically low basal body temperature is more common with hypothyroidism, an underactive thyroid. For a basal temperature, take your temperature after you wake up, before you get out of bed, and before you move around. Typically, basal body temperatures lower than 97.8 to 98.2 degrees Fahrenheit are thought to potentially indicate hypothyroidism. Again, temperature is not conclusive, and doesn't rule out thyroid abnormalities, but it's something you can check right away.

Then there are the various thyroid blood tests.

If you ask your doctor for a thyroid test, in many cases, he'll only do the blood test that measures thyroid-stimulating hormone (TSH). Here's something you need to know. Most labs—and many doctors—have what's called a "normal range" for this test. It runs from around 0.5 to 4.5—so levels above 4.5 are considered "mildly hypothyroid" and levels above 10 are fully hypothyroid. Levels below the normal range may be indicative of hyperthyroidism.

For years, though, doctors have been pussyfooting around this TSH range. Some of the more open-minded doctors say that anything above 2.5 to 3 is already borderline hypothyroid and may warrant treatment. Meanwhile, there are the old stick-in-the-muds who are totally sold on the old numbers. This means, if you are told "your thyroid test was normal," and you don't know the actual number, you could be at 4 or higher, and not get diagnosed or treated.

This is why you MUST ask for the actual numbers, and ask the doctor what he or she considers to be the "normal range." (Remember the doctor who found that my TSH was 7 but said he thought we'd wait a few years until it got up to 10 to treat it?)

But I've also learned that there are other thyroid blood tests that you will want to ask for to help diagnose your hypothyroidism. These include:

- Free T4 (free thyroxine)—Make sure it's the "free" test and not "total." "Free" levels measure the available thyroid hormone and are considered more accurate than the "total" levels. Most of the integrative thyroid experts we talk to like to see this in the upper half of the normal range for optimal function.

- Free T3 (free triiodothyronine)—With this test, they like to see it at least the middle of normal, and many like to see it in the top 25th percentile of the normal range. (Get out your calculators!)

- Reverse T3—This test measures an inactive form of T3 that is produced when the body is under stress. If it's elevated, this can mean that even if the free T3 looks good, the inactive reverse T3 is preventing active T3 from reaching your cells.

- Antithyroid peroxidase (anti-TPO) antibodies—The presence of elevated levels of these antibodies usually indicates Hashimoto's thyroiditis, and if the levels are especially high, that can signal inflammation in the body.

- Thyroid-stimulating immunoglobulins (TSI)—These antibodies are found in as many as 75 to 90 percent of Graves' disease patients. The higher the levels, the more active the Graves' disease is thought to be. The absence of these antibodies does not rule out Graves' disease, however. Some people with autoimmune hypothyroidism can have TSI, which can cause periods of hyperthyroidism.

- Thyroid receptor antibodies (TRAb)—These are seen in most patients with a history of or who currently have Graves' disease. Patients with Graves' disease tend to test positive for a type of TRAb known as stimulatory TRAb.

- Thyroglobulin/thyroid-binding globulin (TBG)—Thyroglobulin, also known as thyroid-binding globulin or TBG, is a protein produced by your thyroid primarily when it is injured or inflamed due to thyroiditis or cancer. When TBG is leaking into the bloodstream and becomes detectable, it indicates some sort of thyroid abnormality. Thyroglobulin is typically elevated in Graves' disease, thyroiditis, and thyroid cancer.

I'll tell you straight out. Most conventional endocrinologists—and believe me, I saw a number of them—are not going to do these tests for you. And many GPs won't either. They are pretty much wedded to the TSH test, and only the TSH test.

This is why, if you suspect a thyroid problem and have symptoms, but a TSH test doesn't show it conclusively, you'll definitely want to make sure you get these additional tests. You may have to hunt around to connect with a good integrative or holistic physician. Or, to get things in motion, you can use a patient-directed lab testing service—Mary and I like MyMedLab—to order the bloodwork yourself, and then take the results to a doctor once you have a better idea of what you're up against.

IMAGING TESTS

In addition to blood tests, a variety of imaging and evaluation tests are sometimes used to make a conclusive diagnosis of thyroid disease, including:

- Nuclear scan or radioactive iodine uptake (RAI-U)—Used to help differentiate between Graves' disease, toxic multinodular goiter, and thyroiditis.
- CT scan—Computer tomography or "CAT scan" is a specialized type of X-ray that is used—not very frequently,

however—to evaluate the thyroid, and frequently to diagnose a goiter or larger nodules.

- Magnetic resonance imaging (MRI)—This test is done when the size and shape of the thyroid need to be evaluated.

- Thyroid ultrasound—Done to evaluate nodules, lumps, and enlargement of your gland. Ultrasound can also determine whether a nodule is a fluid-filled cyst or a mass of solid tissue.

- Needle biopsy or fine-needle aspiration (FNA)—Evaluates suspicious thyroid lumps or thyroid nodules, and assesses whether they are cancerous.

- Afirma Thyroid FNA Analysis (from Veracyte)—A test done on FNA results to conclusively assess nodules for thyroid cancer and to eliminate inconclusive or indeterminate FNA results.

THE DIAGNOSTIC EXAMINATION

In addition to running the full panel of blood tests, and imaging tests as necessary, your doctor should also do a thorough clinical exam. What does that include? Well, first, the doctor needs to put his or her hands on your neck and actually feel your thyroid! When a doctor does this, he or she is looking for lumps or enlargement of your thyroid. Your doctor should also listen to your thyroid with a stethoscope.

The doctor should also check your reflexes—you know, the little hammer on the knee, ankle, and elbow routine. Slow reflexes may point to hypothyroidism, while fast reflexes may signal hyperthyroidism.

The doctor should check your blood pressure and heart rate, because high or very low blood pressure, high or low heart rate, or rhythm irregularities can all be signs of a thyroid problem.

The doctor should also examine your hair and your skin, looking for visible clinical signs of a thyroid condition. In particular, he or she should look for thinning eyebrows at the outer edges, hair loss from head or body, and swelling or puffiness in your hands, feet, or face. The doctor should also look for yellowish, jaundiced skin, blisterlike bumps on the forehead and face, separation of the nail from the nail bed, swollen fingertips, or lesions on the shins—known as pretibial myxedema or dermopathy—which are all more common in hyperthyroidism and Graves' disease.

The doctor should also look at your eyes to check for bulging or protruding eyes, inflamed or dry eyes, eye twitching, and swelling or puffiness in the eyelids.

Finally, the clinical exam should check for enlarged lymph nodes, and the doctor should note if you have any slow movement, tremors, shakiness, slow speech, or hoarseness in your voice.

According to David Borenstein, an integrative physician in New York City:

> For me, a thorough history and physical examination are crucial and will offer a great deal of information. I palpate the thyroid, feeling for enlargement and nodules. I check hair and eyebrows, looking for changes in texture and sparse or bare patches. I check the Achilles reflex, pulse, and blood pressure. I want to hear about symptoms, look for signs of a low thyroid or other hormonal imbalances, and pay particular attention to

such symptoms as fatigue, weight gain, brain fog, swelling, hair loss, brittle nails, and constipation, among others.

I also ask patients about bloating, sugar cravings, and sinus congestion—which are often seen in patients who have underlying yeast overgrowth. I ask about difficulty getting out of bed, higher energy at night, dark circles under the eyes, low blood pressure, exercise intolerance, and salt cravings, which can be signs of an adrenal imbalance. I look for signs and symptoms of perimenopause and insulin resistance. And, of course, family history of thyroid and autoimmune disease in general. It's no longer a surprise to me how many patients tell me that a mother or grandmother had some sort of thyroid disorder.

HYPOTHYROIDISM

We'll start with hypothyroidism, the most common thyroid problem in the United States. People who have had a thyroid surgery or radioactive iodine treatment usually know they're going to become hypothyroid. But the majority of us become hypothyroid as a result of Hashimoto's disease, and so it comes on slowly, and, as in my case, we may not know for years that the thyroid isn't working properly.

Symptoms

We have a detailed risks and symptoms checklist for hypothyroidism at our site for the book, but here's a pretty good list of the common symptoms of hypothyroidism:

You regularly feel extremely exhausted and fatigued.
You often feel depressed, moody, and/or sad.

You're sensitive to cold, and/or you have cold hands and/or feet.

You're gaining weight despite not changing your diet or exercise routine.

You can't lose weight, despite a good diet and exercise.

Your hair is dry, tangled, and/or coarse.

You're losing hair.

You've lost hair from the outer parts of the eyebrows.

You have dry and/or brittle nails.

You have muscle and joint pains and aches.

You have carpal tunnel syndrome or tendinitis in the arms and legs.

The soles of your feet are painful, a condition known as plantar fasciitis.

Your face, eyes, arms, or legs are really swollen or puffy.

You have an unusually low sex drive.

You have unexplained infertility, or recurrent miscarriages with no obvious explanation.

Your menstrual period is heavier than normal, or your period is longer than it used to be or comes more frequently.

You're brain fogged, and your thinking is fuzzy (for example, difficulties with memory and concentration).

You're frequently constipated.

You have a full or sensitive feeling in the neck.

Your voice is raspy or hoarse.

Your heart rate or blood pressure is unusually low.

You have periodic heart palpitations or episodes of atrial fibrillation.

Your total cholesterol and "bad" LDL cholesterol levels are high and may not even respond to diet and medication.

Your allergies have gotten worse, and you experience
symptoms such as itching, prickly hot skin, rashes, and/or
hives (urticaria).
You regularly have infections, including yeast infections, oral
fungus, thrush, or sinus infections.
You feel shortness of breath, sometimes a difficulty drawing a
full breath, or a need to yawn.

Does any of this sound familiar? If you have even a handful of
these symptoms, it's very possible that you might be hypothyroid.

Diagnosis

To diagnose or rule out hypothyroidism, conventional doctors will
typically start with a blood test that measures thyroid-stimulating
hormone (TSH). Some doctors believe that the TSH must be
above 10 to qualify as hypothyroid, and that the level must be
above the top end of the "reference range"—typically, a TSH of
4 or higher—to qualify as subclinical hypothyroidism. Integrative
physicians consider anything above 1 to be potentially suspect, and
they also typically look at low or low-normal free T4 and free T3,
or elevated reverse T3, as signs of possible hypothyroidism.

Hashimoto's thyroiditis is the most common cause of hypothyroidism. The characteristic Hashimoto's thyroiditis patient
has high TSH values and usually low free T3 and T4 thyroid
hormone levels. However, the greatest distinguishing feature for
Hashimoto's is a high concentration of thyroid peroxidase antibodies—known as TPO. Some patients have elevations in antibody levels—along with hypothyroidism symptoms—for months
or years before changes to the TSH, free T4 or free T3 levels are
seen.

Treatment

Once you've been diagnosed with hypothyroidism, what are your treatment options?

Again, I'm going to be straight. The majority of doctors out there will want to give you a drug called levothyroxine. That's the generic name, but the brand names you might recognize: Synthroid, Levothroid, Levoxyl, Unithroid, Tirosint, and Eltroxin. Levothyroxine is a synthetic form of the T4 hormone. (Remember, T4 is the inactive hormone.)

Some people respond to a levothyroxine drug, and do fine on this "T4-only" treatment, but some people don't. In some of us, levothyroxine can even make hair loss worse. And some of the brands have lactose and acacia, which can trigger sensitivities in people who are lactose intolerant or who have pollen allergies. All of the forms of levothyroxine are tablets, except for Tirosint, which is a liquid capsule. Tirosint is hypoallergenic, free of dyes, and apparently helps with absorption for people who have ulcers and stomach issues or who want to drink their coffee at the same time as they take their thyroid medication. (What? You're not supposed to do that? I'll get to that in a minute!)

What about generic levothyroxine? Many people have HMOs or insurance covering their medications, and in that case, you may end up with pharmacies trying to give you generic levothyroxine. And you need to watch out. While generics are fine, when you go to get refills, you can end up getting a batch from any one of the generic levothyroxine manufacturers—and they can vary slightly in potency. So, with each refill, it's sort of Russian roulette. If you find that you can't get stabilized, ask your doctor to prescribe a brand name. If your HMO or insurance won't cover it, and you can afford it, pay for it yourself. It's not very expensive—usually only about $30 a month for a brand name.

Here's something that the doctors probably aren't going to tell you. There are enough studies out there that we can say that the majority of hypothyroid patients feel better not just on a levo-thyroxine drug, but with the addition of the second hormone, T3, in some form—or what they call T4/T3 therapy.

One way to do T4/T3 therapy is simply to add a T3 pill of some type to the levothyroxine treatment. In its generic form, synthetic T3 is called liothyronine. There's a brand name as well, Cytomel. And synthetic T3 is also available by prescription from compounding pharmacies, in a sustained or time-released capsule form.

Natural desiccated thyroid is a drug that was developed in the late 1800s and has been available ever since by prescription. It's made from the desiccated (dried) thyroid gland of pigs, and contains natural forms of T4 and T3, as well as other hormones and nutrients typically found in a thyroid gland. Natural thyroid drugs—which include Armour Thyroid; Nature-Throid, a ge-neric made by Acella in the States; and Erfa (in Canada)—are often considered old-fashioned by endocrinologists, but they've been increasingly popular with more integrative and holistic practitioners. Some patients seem to simply do better on natural thyroid, even compared to an equivalent dose of synthetic T4 and T3. (And I'm one of them!)

After hearing about these options, you are probably wonder-ing which thyroid medication you personally should take for hy-pothyroidism. And there's no magic answer.

Mary always says, "The best thyroid medication is the one that safely works best for you," and I say, amen. Sure, it would be nice if we could say, "Everyone should take this drug, or that drug." But that's not doing anyone any favors.

What works for you may not work for me, and vice versa. And because we're all different, finding the type of medication, brand, combinations, and dosages really is a trial-and-error process. That's why it's so important to have an open-minded doctor who is willing to work with you to find just the right medications, and the right dosages, that work best for you.

I thought it would be helpful for us to share the following chart that summarizes the different forms of thyroid hormone replacement given for hypothyroidism.

PRESCRIPTION THYROID HORMONE REPLACEMENT DRUGS

Generic Name	Brand Name	Description
Levothyroxine	Synthroid, Levoxyl, Levothroid, Unithroid, Eltroxin	Tablet form of synthetic T4. Different brands may have different fillers, dyes, and potential allergens.
Levothyroxine	Tirosint	A manufactured capsule in a liquid, hypoallergenic form of levothyroxine with no fillers or dyes.
Liothyronine	Cytomel	Synthetic T3. Provides the active thyroid hormone.
Liothyronine—SR/TR	Compounded	Synthetic T3, compounded in sustained release or time-release form.
Liotrix	Thyrolar	A combination of synthetic T4/T3 (rarely available commercially).
Natural desiccated thyroid	Nature-Throid, Westhroid, Armour Thyroid, generic in U.S. is from Acella, Erfa (from Canada)	Derived from pigs' thyroids. Includes T4, T3, and other thyroid hormones, including T1 and T2.
Natural desiccated thyroid	Compounded	Natural desiccated thyroid, specially compounded.
Custom-compounded thyroid medication	Compounded	Custom-compounded formulations that may contain synthetic T4, T3, and/or natural desiccated thyroid in various ratios.

HYPERTHYROIDISM

Hyperthyroidism means the thyroid is in overdrive, or overactive, and is producing more thyroid hormone than is necessary. Just as hypothyroidism slows down the body's functioning, hyperthyroidism speeds it up, causing a faster heart rate, higher blood pressure, and a variety of other problems.

Hyperthyroidism is typically caused by the following:

- Autoimmune Graves' disease, which causes the immune system to produce antibodies that bind to the thyroid gland and make it overproduce thyroid hormone
- Autoimmune Hashimoto's disease, which can include spurts of overactivity and hyperthyroidism—shifting back to underactivity, and sometimes back to hyperthyroidism again before eventually slowing down permanently
- A goiter, nodule, or nodules that have caused the thyroid to produce too much thyroid hormone
- Excessive exposure to iodine
- Thyroiditis, an inflammatory condition of the thyroid, which can sometimes make the thyroid overactive
- Being hypothyroid and taking too much thyroid medication

Symptoms

Hyperthyroid patients often have an enlarged thyroid, which can be felt by a doctor upon examination. You may be hyperthyroid if:

- You're rapidly losing weight, or you are eating more and not gaining weight.

- You have insomnia, or you're having a hard time falling asleep or staying asleep.
- You're suffering from anxiety, irritability, nervousness, or even panic attacks.
- You find it difficult to concentrate.
- You're having palpitations, or your pulse and heartbeat are rapid, and blood pressure is elevated.
- You're sweating more than usual, feeling hot when others are not.
- You have hand tremors.
- You're experiencing diarrhea or loose stools.
- You feel tired.
- Your skin is dry, or you may have a thickening of the skin on the shins of your legs.
- Your periods have stopped or are very light and infrequent.
- You're having muscle pain and weakness, especially in the upper arms and thighs.
- You're having eye problems, such as double vision or scratchy eyes, or you notice that your eyes bulge or that more white shows than usual.
- You're having trouble getting pregnant.
- Your hair has become fine and brittle.
- Your behavior or moods are erratic.

Diagnosis

A diagnosis is usually made by administering a thyroid-stimulating hormone (TSH) test. Levels lower than the 0.3 to 0.5 range are considered possibly indicative of hyperthyroidism. High or high-normal total T4/free T4 and/or total T3/free T3 may also indicate hyperthyroidism.

In addition, the thyroid-stimulating immunoglobulin (TSI) and/or thyroid-stimulating antibodies (TSAb) may be measured to diagnose Graves' disease, the autoimmune condition that frequently causes hyperthyroidism.

A radioactive picture of the thyroid may also be taken to see if the thyroid gland is overactive, which is a hallmark of Graves' disease. (Note: Because radioactivity can potentially damage an unborn or breast-feeding baby's thyroid, this test, which requires ingesting [by mouth] radioactive iodine, is not performed on pregnant women or nursing mothers.)

Treating Hyperthyroidism

Sometimes doctors give a beta-blocker—such as atenolol (Tenormin), nadolol (Corgard), metoprolol (Lopressor), or propranolol (Inderal)—to block the effects of thyroid hormone, slow the heart rate, and reduce nervousness and insomnia. These drugs can be useful in rapidly reducing potentially dangerous symptoms until a longer-term thyroid treatment takes effect.

When hyperthyroidism is mild, or occurs in children or young adults, or needs to be promptly controlled (as with elderly patients whose heart disease puts them at risk from the increased heart rate associated with Graves' disease), the treatment is often a course of an antithyroid drug, primarily methimazole, which is known by its brand name Tapazole in the United States. A similar drug, carbimazole, is frequently used outside the States. This drug makes it more difficult for your thyroid to use the iodine it needs to produce thyroid hormone, resulting in a decrease in thyroid hormone. Another antithyroid drug, propylthiouracil

(PTU), is still used by some patients and practitioners, but carries a slightly increased risk of side effects, and so is being used less often.

Antithyroid drugs work for about a third of patients, and taking them for a year to eighteen months may result in a remission in about 40 percent of patients.

A small percentage of patients taking antithyroid drugs have allergic reactions—for example, skin rashes, hives—as well as fever and joint pains. Even less common, but more dangerous, is a decrease in white blood cells that occurs in some people on antithyroid drugs. The risks from antithyroid drugs are highest in the first weeks and months of taking them, and the risks are greater with higher doses of these drugs.

Despite the fact that patients treated with antithyroid drugs may achieve remission, radioactive iodine (RAI) remains the favored treatment of many practitioners in the United States. In RAI, a radioactive iodine drink or pill is given, which delivers the iodine to the thyroid, where the radiation "ablates" the gland, and makes it partially or fully inactive. Most people who have RAI end up hypothyroid for life, and need thyroid hormone replacement treatment.

In the United States, thyroidectomy—a surgery to remove the thyroid gland—is typically done only when the patient cannot tolerate antithyroid drugs or is not a good candidate for RAI (such as a woman who is severely hyperthyroid during pregnancy).

Mary Shomon's book *Living Well with Graves' Disease and Hyperthyroidism* looks at the pros and cons of the various treatments for Graves' disease and also outlines a variety of natural supplements, dietary changes, and lifestyle modifications that may help patients.

GOITER

A goiter is an enlargement of the thyroid. The condition can be detected by ultrasound or X-ray, and may also be diagnosed visually, when the neck is visibly thicker due to the enlarged gland.

The thyroid can become enlarged due to hyperthyroidism, hypothyroidism, autoimmune thyroid disease, multiple goiters, or inflammation from thyroiditis. It can also become enlarged due to deficiency or overconsumption of iodine.

Symptoms

The signs of a goiter are:

- Enlarged thyroid, a swollen-looking or -feeling neck
- The neck or thyroid area is tender to the touch
- A tight feeling in the throat
- Frequent coughing
- A hoarse voice
- Difficulty swallowing
- Difficulty breathing and shortness of breath, especially at night
- A feeling that food is getting stuck in your throat

Goiter can be caused by autoimmune conditions, as well as imbalances in iodine levels. If you have too much iodine exposure (for example, from taking a heart medication such as amiodarone), you might end up with excess thyroid hormone and a goiter. If there is insufficient iodine in your diet, a hypothyroid goiter can develop. The use of iodized salt has wiped out the majority of goiters from iodine deficiency in the United States, but 10 to 20 percent of goiters in the United States are still due to iodine deficiency, and iodine-deficiency goiter outside the U.S. is still common

Diagnosis

One way to detect a goiter is a "thyroid neck check." See page 83 for instructions on how to perform this simple self-test. These steps can be involved in diagnosing goiter:

- A doctor's examination to observe neck enlargement
- A blood test to determine if your thyroid is producing irregular amounts of thyroid hormone
- An antibody test to confirm an autoimmune disease, which may be the cause of your goiter
- An ultrasound test to evaluate the size of the enlargement
- A radioactive isotope thyroid scan to produce an image of the thyroid and provide visual information about the nature of the thyroid enlargement

Treating Goiter

Treatment for goiter depends on how enlarged the thyroid has become as well as other symptoms. Treatments can include:

- Observation and monitoring, which is typically done if your goiter is not large and is not causing symptoms or thyroid dysfunction
- Medications, including thyroid hormone replacement, which can help shrink your goiter, or aspirin or corticosteroid drugs to shrink thyroid inflammation
- Surgery if the goiter is very large, continues to grow while on thyroid hormone, or symptoms continue, or if

the goiter is in a dangerous location (e.g., the windpipe or esophagus) or is cosmetically unsightly. If the goiter contains suspicious nodules, this may also be reason for surgery.

THYROID NODULES

Sometimes your thyroid gland has lumps, also known as nodules. These nodules, which can be solid or liquid-filled, are called toxic nodules when they are overactive and produce far too much thyroid hormone. When there are a lot of them, the condition is referred to as a toxic multinodular goiter. When nodules overproduce hormone, it may result in hyperthyroidism. Some nodules do not produce any hormone at all, or may impair the gland's ability to produce thyroid hormone, and thus contribute to hypothyroidism. Thyroid nodules are fairly common. An estimated 1 in 12 to 15 women and 1 in 50 men has a thyroid nodule. More than 90 percent of nodules are benign (except in pregnant women, in whom approximately 27 percent of nodules are typically cancerous). It's vital to have your doctor examine any nodule as soon as you notice it.

Symptoms

Symptoms of thyroid nodules include palpitations, insomnia, weight loss, anxiety, and tremors, which are all common in hyperthyroidism as well. Nodules can also trigger hypothyroidism, and symptoms might include weight gain, fatigue, and depression. Some people will cycle back and forth between hyperthyroid and hypothyroid symptoms. Others may have difficulty swallowing, feelings of fullness, pain or pressure in the neck, a hoarse voice, and neck tenderness. Many people have nodules with no obvious symptoms related to thyroid dysfunction at all.

Diagnosis

Nodules are usually evaluated by:

- A blood test to determine whether they are producing thyroid hormone
- A radioactive thyroid scan, which looks at the reaction of the nodule to small amounts of radioactive material
- An ultrasound of the thyroid to determine whether the nodule is solid or fluid-filled
- A fine-needle aspiration or needle biopsy of the nodules to determine whether they may be cancerous

Treating Thyroid Nodules

Depending on the results of the evaluation, nodules may be left alone and monitored periodically, assuming they aren't causing serious difficulty, treated with thyroid hormone replacement to help shrink them, or surgically removed if they are causing problems with breathing or if test results indicate a malignancy. Some endocrinologists are also treating some nodules with percutaneous ethanol injections (PEI) and ultrasound, to shrink the nodules without surgery.

THYROID CANCER

In the United States, thyroid cancer is on the rise and is the fastest-growing cancer, with more than 45,000 new cases diagnosed each year. Thyroid cancer is for the most part considered very treatable, but the incidence of thyroid cancer has increased substantially in the past decade, and experts believe it's in part due to exposure to radiation.

The treatment and prognosis for thyroid cancer depends on the type. Papillary and follicular thyroid cancers are the most common types; an estimated 80 to 90 percent of all thyroid cancers fall into this category. Most of these cancers can be treated successfully when discovered early. Medullary thyroid carcinoma (MTC) makes up 5 to 10 percent of all thyroid cancers. If discovered before it metastasizes to other parts of the body, it has a good cure rate. There are two types of medullary thyroid cancer: sporadic and familial. Anyone with a family history of MTC should have blood tests to measure calcitonin levels, which may indicate a strong possibility of a genetic predisposition. If found, a thyroidectomy may be performed as a preventive measure. Anaplastic thyroid carcinoma is quite rare, accounting for only 1 to 2 percent of all thyroid cancers. It tends to be quite aggressive and is the least likely to respond to typical methods of treatment, though new drug treatments are showing some promise with this most difficult form of thyroid cancer.

Symptoms

Although many patients are asymptomatic at first, possible symptoms of thyroid cancer include:

- A lump in the neck
- Changes in the voice
- Difficulty in breathing or swallowing
- Lymph node swelling

Diagnosis

The main diagnostic procedure for suspected thyroid cancer is a fine-needle aspiration (FNA) biopsy of the thyroid nodule. Using a needle, fluid and cells are removed from various parts of all nodules that can be felt, and these samples are evaluated. Frequently, FNA tests are done with an ultrasound machine to help guide the needle into nodules that are too small to be felt. Between 60 and 80 percent of FNA tests show that the nodule is benign. Only about 1 in 20 FNA tests reveals cancer. If a case is classified as suspicious, a surgical biopsy may be needed. If an FNA result is inconclusive or indeterminate, a newer test process, called Afirma Thyroid Analysis, from Veracyte can conclusively diagnose or rule out thyroid cancer, preventing an unnecessary thyroidectomy.

In everyone except pregnant women, a radioactive thyroid scan is frequently done in order to identify if the nodules are "cold," meaning they have a greater potential to be cancerous.

Treating Thyroid Cancer

There are three key treatments for patients with cancer of the thyroid. The following types are commonly used:

- Surgery (removal of the thyroid and the cancer)
- Radiation therapy (to kill remaining cancer cells)
- Hormone therapy (to stop cancer cells from growing)

Surgery is the most common treatment of thyroid cancer. A doctor may remove the cancer using one of the following operations:

- Lobectomy removes only the side of the thyroid where the cancer is found. Lymph nodes in the area may be taken out (biopsied) to see if they contain cancer.
- Near-total thyroidectomy removes all of the thyroid except for a small part.
- Total thyroidectomy removes the entire thyroid.
- Lymph node dissection removes lymph nodes in the neck that contain cancer.

Radiation for cancer of the thyroid may come from a machine outside the body (external radiation therapy), but most commonly from a pill or liquid form of radioactive iodine (RAI). Because the thyroid takes up iodine, the radioactive iodine collects in any thyroid tissue remaining in the body and kills any remaining cancer cells.

After removal of the gland—and radiation—patients typically end up hypothyroid for the rest of their lives, and must take thyroid replacement hormone. In some cases, "suppression" is also part of the thyroid cancer follow-up—this means that the thyroid hormone replacement medication must be at a dosage to keep TSH levels low—or undetectable at close to 0, in some patients—to help prevent a relapse of cancer.

Overall, the prognosis for thyroid cancer is quite good. However, survivors need to be vigilant in case of a reccurrence. Regular checkups and periodic scans by their physicians are necessary to monitor for recurrence and ensure proper thyroid hormone replacement.

RELATED CONDITIONS

There are some conditions that you should know about, as they are more common in people with thyroid disease. While the connections aren't always understood, if you have a thyroid condition, you'll want to be aware of the symptoms and the increased risk of your developing these conditions. Similarly, if you have any of these conditions, keep in mind that you should periodically be evaluated for autoimmune thyroid disease.

- Epstein-Barr virus (EBV) and mononucleosis
- Carpal tunnel syndrome
- Tarsal tunnel syndrome—an inflammation/irritation/ weakness of the shin/lower leg area similar to carpal tunnel
- Tendinitis
- Plantar fasciitis—a painful inflammatory condition of the foot that causes pain on the underside of the heel
- Polycystic ovary syndrome (PCOS)
- Mitral valve prolapse (MVP)—a heart murmur that can cause heart palpitations or skipped beats
- Down syndrome
- Depression, bipolar disease, panic disorder, panic attacks, generalized anxiety disorder
- Iron-deficiency anemia
- Hemochromatosis—a condition of excess iron that can cause cirrhosis of the liver, adrenal insufficiency, heart failure, and/or diabetes
- Urticaria (hives)
- Endometriosis

- Candidiasis/yeast overgrowth
- Chronic fatigue syndrome and fibromyalgia
- Type 1 diabetes
- Metabolic syndrome/insulin resistance/type 2 diabetes
- High cholesterol/hyperlipidemia
- Other autoimmune diseases, i.e., multiple sclerosis, rheumatoid arthritis, lupus, psoriasis, pernicious anemia, alopecia, vitiligo, etc.
- Adrenal diseases: Addison's disease, Cushing's disease

5

Thyroid Treatment Challenges

The journey of a thousand miles must begin with a single step.
—LAO TZU

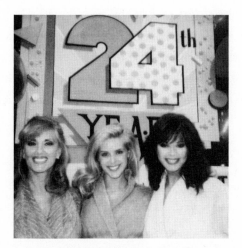

On the set of The Price Is Right,
with Janice Pennington and Holly Hallstrom

So there you have it. Thyroid in a nutshell. Sounds easy, right? But it's not. I'm living proof, going years without tests, and even then having to fight to get treated and then having to find the right treatment. And after seventeen years as a patient advocate, Mary has heard every story in the book about the seemingly insurmountable odds some people have faced to get diagnosed and treated.

Here are some of the challenges you might come up against,

and some tips and advice to help you face those challenges head-on and prevail!

THYROID TESTING

Always Ask for a Thyroid Peroxidase Antibodies (TPO) as Part of Your Initial Panel

I have to wonder, years ago, when I was exhausted, depressed, and gaining weight, if one of the many doctors I consulted had done a thyroid peroxidase antibodies (TPO) test, would they have found my Hashimoto's disease? If they had, I might have been able to get treatment and avoid years of struggling with poor health. I don't want to think about that too much, or I might cry, to be honest.

Don't make the same mistake! If you suspect you might be hypothyroid, and the doctor offers to run a TSH test, you really ought to insist that they add in the TPO test as well. If the TPO antibodies are elevated, that can tell you that your thyroid is already in the process of self-destruction.

And boy does it frost me to hear that there are studies that show that treating elevated thyroid antibodies, even in the presence of normal TSH levels, may help resolve symptoms, and often prevent development of full hypothyroidism.

Don't accept the excuse that Mary's first endocrinologist gave her when Mary requested an antibodies test and that doctor refused. "Why bother?" the doctor said. "All we can do is treat hypothyroidism, we can't treat the autoimmune disease."

There you have it. That's the conventional endocrinology view of autoimmune disease—they can't even be bothered because they have nothing they believe can help.

That doesn't make sense. There are studies that show that even low-dose treatment of people who have "normal" levels but elevated antibodies may keep them from becoming fully hypothyroid, and keep antibodies from going up. But it seems the endocrinologists haven't read those studies, for some reason.

And beyond that, the truth is, if you have an autoimmune disease, you need to know, because it means your family members—like siblings, parents, and children—are also at an increased risk for autoimmune conditions. And we are also starting to learn about various things you can actually do—like going gluten free, for example, or taking selenium—that may help calm inflammation and reduce antibodies, not to mention help us feel better. So don't take no for an answer, and make sure they run that TPO test.

Push for a Reverse T3 Test

Even though some doctors will look at you cross-eyed when you ask for it, you will want to ask for the reverse T3 test as well. If they don't have any idea what the test is, or they tell you they don't do it, it's time to move on to a new doctor.

It's a really important test. Oakland, California, area holistic gynecologist and hormone expert Sara Gottfried, MD, has integrated reverse T3 testing into her practice. "I used to order reverse T3 in a patient if I'd optimized the TSH and free T3, but the patient still had hypothyroidism symptoms. Now I order it more often at the start, because I think it's informative in deciding about the treatment formulation. For example, if a patient has high reverse T3, I'm more likely to use the compounded, time-released T3 as part of their treatment."

The reverse T3 test helps detect if you don't have enough active T3 hormone reaching your cells. That can happen because you're not converting T4 to T3 properly, there are nutritional issues, or you're under a great deal of stress.

Reverse T3 is another one of those tests that you can order yourself if you need to, but you'll need a sharp practitioner who knows what to do with the results.

Don't Just Accept "Your TSH Is Normal"

Many of you have already asked for a thyroid test, had it run, and gotten "the call." You know the call. Someone from the doctor's office leaves you a quick voice mail that says, "your thyroid tests were normal."

Don't accept this!!!

Call back and tell them that you want to know the actual number and the reference range. Better yet, ask for a hard copy to be faxed, emailed, or mailed to you, so that you can look at it. That way, you'll be able to determine exactly where you are.

Remember, there are many doctors out there who are still using outdated guidelines for TSH tests, and so if your TSH is 3.5, or 4, or 4.5, those doctors will say you're "normal" when other doctors would say that you're hypothyroid.

Push for Free T3 Testing and T3 Treatment When Needed

Even after I was first diagnosed, I spent awhile just dragging myself around taking a levothyroxine drug. It just wasn't doing it for me, and I was still dealing with a laundry list of thyroid symptoms. If I had pushed to have my free T3 tested, it would have shown how low the level was. And that was something that could have, and should have, been treated. But it wasn't . . . until I finally got to the naturopath who understood that.

Some people do beautifully when a T3 medication—like Cytomel or time-release compounded T3—is added to the levothyroxine. I wouldn't know if that might have worked for me, because my doctors never offered it, and I didn't know to ask back then. But luckily, my naturopath tested my free T3, saw it was low, and offered me the option of natural desiccated thyroid.

Make Sure Your Treatment Is Optimized

Most thyroid patients end up hypothyroid. Mary sometimes says, "with thyroid disease, all roads lead to hypothyroidism." And what this means is that ultimately, treatments for thyroid problems often result in ablating or removing the thyroid, or otherwise slowing it down or making a person hypothyroid. Whether it's surgery for thyroid cancer or goiter, antithyroid drugs for hyperthyroidism, radioactive iodine (RAI) treatment, or the gradual destruction of the thyroid in Hashimoto's disease, most thyroid patients ultimately end up hypothyroid and taking thyroid hormone replacement medication.

Conventional doctors will tell you, as they told me, that a levothyroxine (T4) drug—like Synthroid or Levoxyl—is the only treatment, the best treatment, the safest treatment, or whatever other superlative they feel like applying that day. But the truth is that patients respond differently to different brands, different medications, and different combinations. I know that I certainly did, as did Mary. The key is working with a doctor who recognizes that and is willing to go through a process of trial and error to help you find out what works best for you.

Many conventional doctors are just diehards—they always start out with a levothyroxine drug. Some practitioners like to start with a T4 drug but will add T3 if needed and switch to a natural thyroid drug as a third option. Others may prefer to start with natural thyroid.

Whatever you start taking, the key is to keep track of your symptoms and test results, so that you can decide over time whether you might benefit from changing brands, changing medications, or adjusting your dose.

Dr. Kevin Passero, a Washington, D.C.–based naturopathic physician, explains how open-minded physicians view thyroid hormone replacement:

> Through my years of experience, I have learned there is no one answer to this question. In order to have the best outcomes, every person needs to be evaluated on a case by case basis. In my early years, I might have said that natural desiccated thyroid drugs like Armour Thyroid and Nature-Throid were the best, and standard prescriptions like Synthroid were less ideal, but I have learned that these views do not reflect what plays out in clinical practice. I will say that the majority of people with hypothyroidism have only been prescribed the most common thyroid medication, Synthroid, and feel there is something to be desired. I agree wholeheartedly and find that the majority of these people often need that prescription augmented or changed entirely to feel their best. With that said, I have met many patients that thrive on Synthroid and other synthetic T4 analogues, and I have learned to take an approach that always puts the patient's needs first and removes any predetermined bias on my part.

In my own case, I didn't really feel like I was back on track to feeling well until I went to a naturopathic physician and switched to a natural desiccated thyroid drug. After a few years taking Synthroid, going to natural thyroid was a dramatic—and welcome—change for me.

In Mary's case, she spent a number of years trying different medications with her physician—she started on synthetic levothyroxine, then switched to a T4/T3 synthetic combo drug, Thyrolar. (You can't get it much anymore.) Then she went to levothyroxine plus a separate T3 drug. Eventually she switched to Armour Thyroid, and then after Armour reformulated, she switched to Nature-Throid, and her doctor added in a small amount of compounded time-release T3. If it sounds complicated, it is . . . but the most important thing is having an open-minded doctor who is willing to work with you to help you feel well and knows how to safely prescribe the different thyroid medications until you find the right combination for you. Mary's been on her current mix of thyroid medications for more than five years, and it's been working well for her.

Here are a few pointers that may be of help in optimizing your treatment.

First, the various thyroid drugs have different fillers, dyes, and binders, and you may be sensitive to some of these ingredients. Consider trying a different brand if you react poorly. (Note: one of the things many patients don't know is that Synthroid contains lactose and acacia, common allergens, and some patients find that switching to another brand can help.) The Tirosint capsule form of levothyroxine has no fillers, binders, or dyes, and it's totally hypoallergenic, so it's an option if you have allergies and sensitivities.

Second, some patients seem to need additional T3, and studies suggest that the majority of patients feel better with a T4/

T3 combination treatment, than a T4-only treatment. Others are extremely sensitive to T3, and do well on T4-only treatment. Talk to your doctor about which drug, combination, and brand is best for you.

Third, some patients who are unable to get relief of symptoms with synthetic drugs—including T4/T3 combinations—do better on natural desiccated thyroid drugs.

If you are still suffering from thyroid symptoms despite being treated, it's likely that your treatment is not optimized. *Optimized* is a term that patients—and integrative practitioners—use to say that it's not enough just to get thyroid medication. You need the right amount and type of medication, in order to notice improvement in your symptoms.

So what does *optimized* mean? Mary has surveyed some of the top integrative hormone experts around the country, and they believe that the optimal TSH level for the majority of thyroid patients is a TSH between 1 and 2. They feel that the free T4 levels should be in the top half of the normal range, and the free T3 levels in the top half at minimum—and in many cases the top 25 percent—of the normal range. Reverse T3 should not be substantially elevated.

Oakland, California, area holistic gynecologist and hormone expert Dr. Sara Gottfried, author of *The Hormone Cure,* focuses on two key optimization goals for her thyroid patients: improving symptoms such as fatigue, weight gain, hair loss, etc., by at least 80 percent, and targeting a TSH of between 0.3 and 1.0 and free T3 in the top half of the normal range.

Says Dr. Gottfried:

Not all my patients can tolerate such an aggressive goal with TSH, but I find that range is often the sweet spot. Another key aspect of optimization is that the adrenal function, meaning cortisol and DHEA-S, are in the normal range. So many of my hypothyroid patients also have adrenal dysregulation, and don't feel better on thyroid augmentation unless their adrenals are optimized simultaneously.

In our patient/physician partnership, we optimize most readily when a patient is primed for focus on all things thyroid: she is studying up, taking her supplements, addressing her adrenal issues . . . but optimization often is hardest in women with autoimmune thyroiditis—there we have to work not only on the endocrine system but on quieting the immune system as well.

In our support communities, we hear all the time from patients whose doctors put them on thyroid medication, leave them with a TSH of 4.5, and declare them "treated." That's ridiculous!

What happens is that some people simply aren't getting enough T4 or T3 medication. And integrative doctors believe that there are also many of us who have problems converting T4 to T3, or whose cells don't absorb T3 effectively.

The whole T3 issue is a hot button. Remember that T3 is the active thyroid hormone, and when everything is working fine, the body will properly convert T4 to T3. But if you have nutritional deficiencies, toxic exposures, or autoimmunity, that conversion process can go awry, leaving hypothyroid. In late 2009, there was a Danish study published in the respected *European Journal of Endocrinology*. The study looked at the effects of a levothyroxine-only therapy versus levothyroxine plus T3. They used a fairy small dose of 20 mcg of T3 for the study. They evaluated the quality of life, energy, depression, and other mental health symptoms at the start, then put half of them on T4/T3 combo, and the other half on T4 only (but the patients didn't know which they were on). At the twelve-week point, they were evaluated again, switched to the opposite medication for twelve weeks, and then a final evaluation was done.

The study showed that among the patients, most of whom were women, while nearly half preferred the combination treatment, only 15 percent preferred the levothyroxine-only treatment. This is what we hear from the patient community as well. Many people who get to try a T4/T3 combination prefer that over T4 only.

You do want to keep in mind that people—especially those with heart issues—may find T3 too stimulating to heart rate and pulse, or may have palpitations when taking some forms of T3. If these patients are going to continue taking T3, some doctors will prescribe a time-release T3 from a compounding pharmacy.

There's also the issue of natural desiccated thyroid. This drug known as porcine thyroid—or "natural thyroid" or "pig thyroid"—is manufactured from the dried thyroid gland of pigs. The drugs in this category include Armour Thyroid, Nature-throid, Erfa Thyroid, and the generic from Acella. Natural thyroid is not available over-the-counter, nor is it the same as glandular supplements. It is an FDA-regulated prescription medication.

Remember that conventional endocrinology doesn't have much use for T3 and natural thyroid. Endocrinologists often say that no one needs T3—"everyone converts T4 into T3" is a popular myth you hear from the endos. And as for natural desiccated thyroid drugs, they often say it's "old-fashioned" or "inconsistent," and then they refuse to prescribe it. That's why so many of us end up with holistic or integrative physicians, or naturopathic doctors, who have a more open-minded view of diagnosing and treating thyroid issues, especially hypothyroidism, and who don't have a cookie-cutter, one-size-fits-all approach to treatment.

Naturopathic physician Dr. Kevin Passero explains:

> There are many different types of thyroid medication available as well as natural treatments for certain thyroid conditions, and different people need different ones in order to thrive. The biggest problem with traditional thyroid care is that it is approached as a one-size-fits-all condition. Nothing could be further from the truth when it comes to working with thyroid disorders. A holistic/integrative approach to thyroid dysfunction is essential for most people to have optimal outcomes.

OTHER ADVICE AND IDEAS

Seasonally Adjust Your Thyroid Dosage

One thing I didn't know about until recently is that temperature changes can affect the thyroid dosage you need. Here in Arizona, it's warm year-round, but those of you who have hot summers and cold winters (like I used to have back in Minnesota!) may need a seasonal dosage adjustment. We tend to need slightly more thyroid medication when it's cold, and slightly less when it's warm. Some doctors will even issue a standing order for a dosage adjustment when the seasons change. But if you don't know if you are having seasonal fluctuations, plan to get tested at least twice in a year—when winter starts and when summer starts—to see if you're having any fluctuations, and if any changes are needed to your dosage.

Take Your Medication Properly

Sure, we all get those inserts with the tiny print every time we pick up a prescription. But you know what? No one tells us some of the most important things you need to know in order to get the most possible benefit out of thyroid medication and to properly absorb it. But I'm going to tell you!

- You're not going to like this, but you should wait an hour after taking your thyroid medication before you drink your morning coffee. That goes for decaf too. There are acids in coffee that can interfere with proper absorption. (If you're taking Tirosint, however, they've found that coffee doesn't interfere with its absorption.)
- Don't take your thyroid hormone medication within four hours of taking calcium supplements, like Tums or Mylanta, tablets or liquid form. This also goes for calcium-fortified orange juice, which has become very popular.
- Don't take thyroid hormone medication within four hours of taking any supplements that contain iron. Remember that prenatal vitamins almost always contain iron!
- Try to take your thyroid hormone around the same time each day. For best results, doctors recommend taking it in the morning on an empty stomach, about an hour before eating.
- If you start or stop a high-fiber diet while you are on thyroid hormone, have your thyroid function retested around eight weeks after you've changed your diet. A high-fiber diet can change your absorption. This is not a reason to avoid high-fiber foods, but any correlation is something to check.

- If you start or stop an antidepressant medication, or a medication that contains estrogen—like the Pill or hormone replacement therapy (HRT)—have your thyroid levels retested around eight weeks later. These drugs can affect absorption, so you may need a change in your dosage.

Consider Changing How You Take Your Medication

If you are taking a levothyroxine drug, there is no proven benefit to taking your thyroid medication multiple times a day. But if you're taking a drug that includes T3 (like Cytomel, or the natural desiccated thyroid drugs), talk to the doctor about whether you should split the dose. Some people take their initial dose in the morning and a second dose in the afternoon or evening, to help maintain a more steady level of T3.

There are also some studies that have shown that people who take their full dosage of levothyroxine at night—instead of first thing in the morning—may have better absorption. So you may want to talk to your doctor about whether to take your thyroid medication at night. Another side benefit: you can have a cup of coffee as soon as you wake up, and there's no need to wait to take iron or calcium supplements in the morning.

Remember . . . you should always discuss any change in the way you take your medication with your physician.

Don't Refuse to or Forget to Take Your Medication!

Finally, don't forget to take your medication. I'm always surprised by how many fellow thyroid patients say they forget to take their thyroid medication—or the number of those who are prescribed medication but don't feel like taking it!

When you are taking thyroid hormone replacement, it's critical that you take it every day as prescribed. Even missing a day or two can really throw things out of whack, and you could be paying for it with weeks of feeling bad. If you have trouble remembering, try putting a reminder into your smartphone, leave your thyroid pill next to your toothbrush, the coffeepot, or on top of your alarm clock, or put a reminder note somewhere you'll always see it every morning, like the refrigerator or your bathroom mirror.

Make Sure Other Medications Aren't Interfering with or Interacting with Your Thyroid Medication

Many thyroid patients aren't aware that certain antidepressants—especially sertraline (Zoloft), paroxetine (Paxil), and fluoxetine (Prozac)—may interfere with the effectiveness of thyroid hormone replacement medication. That's not a reason not to take these medications, but if you're on thyroid treatment, and you start or stop an antidepressant, or vice versa, make sure you get rechecked, and make sure all the doctors know about the prescribed antidepressants and thyroid medications.

You should also know that there are other drugs that interact with your thyroid medication, become stronger or weaker when taken with thyroid medication, or affect your thyroid function. This is not an all-inclusive list, but some of the drugs to keep in mind are:

- Insulin
- Cholesterol-lowering drugs cholestyramine or colestipol— these drugs bind thyroid hormones. Some brand names are

Colestrol, Questran, Colestid. Make sure you leave at least four to five hours between taking them and your thyroid medications.

- Anticoagulants ("blood thinners")—these include Warfarin, Coumadin, and Heparin
- Corticosteroids/adrenocorticosteroids—brands include Cortisone, Cortistab, and Cortone
- Amiodarone HCL—the heart drug known by the brand name Cordarone
- Ketamine—an anesthetic, and also a popular illegal drug used as a recreational hallucinogen known as "K" or "Special K"
- Theophylline—an asthma drug
- Lithium—used to treat bipolar disease and some forms of depression
- Phenytoin—an anticonvulsant; a well-known brand is Dilantin
- Carbamazepine—an anticonvulsant pain medicine; a popular brand is Tegretol
- Rifampin—an antituberculosis medication

FOCUS ON NUTRITION AND VITAMINS

You definitely want to make sure that you're getting proper nutrition to support your thyroid. Most of us don't get all the vitamins, minerals, and amino acids we need from food, so you will probably want to include at least some supplements. A few basics:

A good, high-potency multivitamin is really helpful for thyroid patients. Look for one that has high amounts of vitamins B,

C, and E and a good range of minerals, including zinc, but not too much iodine. Specifically, you want to make sure your vitamin includes the following thyroid essentials:

- Vitamin A helps produce thyroid hormone.
- Vitamin B_2 (riboflavin) helps endocrine function.
- Vitamin B_3 (niacin) helps energy reach cells.
- Vitamin B_6 (pyridoxine) helps the body convert iodine to thyroid hormone.
- Vitamin B_{12} (cyanocobalamin, methylcobalamin) helps counteract hypothyroidism-related B12 deficiency.
- Vitamin E is a potent antioxidant and also helps with immune function.
- Vitamin C. You may want to add some extra vitamin C. Many experts recommend as much as 2,000 to 3,000 mg of vitamin C each day. You can use capsules or powdered forms of vitamin C. It can help the immune system, and there's also research that shows better absorption of thyroid medication when it's taken along with vitamin C.
- Vitamin D. Even down here in sunny Arizona, many people are deficient in vitamin D. Between avoiding the sun, sunscreens, and not eating or drinking many vitamin D–fortified foods, most of us are deficient in D. And now we know that D is not only a vitamin but a hormone, and that it's needed for the pituitary gland to produce thyroid hormone. It also plays a role in T4 to T3 conversion and immune health. You definitely need to have vitamin D levels checked, and supplement them if they're low. What's low? Many of the integrative doctors we hear from like to

see vitamin D in the 50 to 80 range (where 100 is the top end of the normal range).

- Probiotics are supplements that contain live bacteria: the "good" bacteria found in fermented foods such as miso and dairy products such as yogurt and some cheeses. We are meant to have good bacteria in sufficient quantities in our intestinal system, because they help digestion and boost the immune system. To get enough probiotics, you'll probably want to take a daily supplement.

- Selenium is a particularly important mineral for thyroid function. It helps with T4-to-T3 conversion. Selenium supplementation has been shown to reduce inflammation in patients with autoimmune thyroiditis. But be careful, because too much selenium can be toxic. Your total intake of selenium from all sources—multivitamin and additional supplements—should not exceed 400 micrograms per day. Note: that's mcg and NOT milligrams/mg.

- Zinc is crucial for thyroid hormone production and conversion, and can also help keep T3 levels from dropping.

- L-tyrosine is an amino acid needed for the creation and release of thyroid hormone. It is a common ingredient in thyroid support supplements.

- Essential fatty acids (EFAs) are nutrients, found in certain kinds of fats, that the body cannot produce. The key essential fatty acids include omega-3/alpha-linolenic acid (ALA); eicosapentaenoic acid (EPA); docosahexaenoic acid (DHA), found in fresh fish—such as mackerel, tuna, herring, flounder, sardines, salmon, rainbow trout, bass—from cold, deep oceans; as well as in linseed oil, flaxseeds, black currant and pumpkin seeds, cod liver oil, shrimp, oysters, leafy greens, soybeans, walnuts, wheat germ, fresh sea vegetables such as seaweed, and fish oil. The other important EFA is omega-6/linoleic acid/gamma-linolenic acid (GLA), found in breast milk, sesame, safflower, cotton, sunflower seeds and oil, corn and corn oil, soybeans, raw nuts, legumes, leafy greens, black currant seeds, evening primrose oil, borage oil, spirulina, soybeans, and lecithin. EFAs can help reduce inflammation, help with metabolizing fats, positively improve blood sugar and cholesterol levels, and help keep hair, skin, and nails healthy. In addition to adding EFA-rich foods to your diet, you can also use supplements, including fish oil supplements. Go for the ones that are free of toxins, and "burpless." You can't go wrong with a few of the key brands, like Carlson's, Barlean's, and Enzymatic Therapies. Evening primrose and borage oil are rich in GLA, and may also help with skin and hair.

Watch Goitrogens

Goitrogens are products and foods that promote goiter—an enlarged thyroid—and can slow the thyroid. If you're hypothyroid because you've had your thyroid surgically removed, you don't have to worry about goitrogens. But if you still have a thyroid, you have to be careful not to overdo it with the raw goitrogens. (The good news is, cooking or steaming can usually deactivate most of the problem.)

One thing in particular to be careful about—raw smoothies and juicing. That healthy drink you're making could be filled with raw veggies that will slow your thyroid!

The following list contains some of the more common and potent goitrogens:

African cassava

Babassu (palm-tree fruit from Brazil and Africa)

Broccoli

Brussels sprouts

Cabbage

Cauliflower

Kale

Kohlrabi

Millet

Mustard

Radishes

Rutabaga

Turnips

Watercress

Be Careful with Soy

There's a great deal of controversy about soy. You hear how healthy it is, and many popular diet shakes are chock-full of soy. At the same time, some experts are concerned because soy can have hormonal effects in the body. It's also a common allergen, and much of it is genetically modified. Keep in mind that soy is a goitrogen, and it can also interfere with absorption of thyroid medication.

If you no longer have your thyroid, some soy food is probably fine for you. Try to avoid processed and genetically modified soy— choose soy products that specifically say "organic, non-GMO." Also, be careful about consuming high levels of soy, because even in the absence of a thyroid gland, soy binds to thyroid hormone and can reduce the effectiveness of your medication.

If you still have a thyroid gland, you'll want to be careful about using too much soy, especially soy pills, powders, and supplements. Daily overconsumption of too much soy may contribute to the worsening of your thyroid problem. Some experts suggest that you limit soy to the purest forms, like tofu and tempeh, and avoid edamame and soy milk.

Eliminate Gluten

My friend Janell has celiac disease, so I've been familiar with the gluten-free diet for years. But I didn't realize that celiac disease and gluten intolerance, which make it difficult or impossible to digest wheat and gluten products, can trigger autoimmune disease and can make autoimmune symptoms worse.

In my case, testing showed that I had some food intolerances, and in particular, I was sensitive to wheat and gluten. Dr. Christianson recommended that I follow the gluten-free diet.

Here's what he said:

In someone like Gena, when you introduce wheat and gluten products, the immune system activates and goes on the attack. So eliminating these foods from the diet can help calm a hyperimmune, hyperinflammatory state.

For me, gut health is crucial, and it's a key area to focus on for many autoimmune patients. Two-thirds of our immune system is in the gut, as it's our first and main point of entry. If we don't have a healthy lining, and a balance of flora, the body starts attacking large, undigested, naturally occurring proteins, and we see people getting sensitized to more and more items, leading to allergies, autoimmunity, inflammation, and even environmental sensitivities.

You can have a test to determine if you have actual celiac disease—the antigliadin antibodies blood test can pick up on many cases of gluten and wheat sensitivity. In some cases, they want to do an endoscopic biopsy to confirm celiac disease. Even if the tests are negative, I know that in my case and Mary's, and for many of the patients we hear from, going gluten free has helped with weight loss, fatigue, bloating, and energy, so it may be worth giving it a try for a few months to see if it helps.

Be Careful with Iodine

Iodine is a hot topic in the thyroid world. Some practitioners say everyone with a thyroid problem needs iodine, and others warn that giving some thyroid patients iodine is like throwing gasoline on a fire. Whom do we believe?

My doctor, Alan Christianson, calls iodine the "Goldilocks of medicine," because for many patients, it's too high, or too low, and for the thyroid to function, it needs to be just right.

It seems that the key is knowing if you need iodine, and if so, making sure you take it in the best possible form. The best way to evaluate your iodine levels is with the urinary iodine clearance test. Your integrative doctor can get this test kit for you, or you can order one yourself in most parts of the country. This test measures your body's need for iodine. If you come back as iodine deficient, and your practitioner recommends it, you may want to try iodine supplementation. Typically, the best form combines both iodine and iodide and is found in a pill format known as Iodoral, or a liquid called Lugol's solution.

Some practitioners and patients have found that, even if tests show an iodine deficiency, iodine supplements still aggravate their thyroid symptoms. Mary, for example, can't take any iodine supplements. It makes her thyroid inflamed, and she feels exhausted and achy within a day or two of starting. She's worked around it by making sure that she regularly includes some iodine-rich foods—like seaweed salads and shrimp—in her diet, and that seems to work for her.

Optimize Ferritin Levels

Ferritin is the protein that stores and releases iron into the bloodstream. It's crucial for thyroid function, hormone balance, and maintaining energy, and low ferritin is often an issue if you're going through hair loss.

Many practitioners recommend that ferritin levels should be between 50 and 80 (on a scale where 100 is the top end of normal) for hormones to function. You can raise ferritin with food—for meat-eaters, grass-fed red meat is a good source—and vegetable sources include kale, chard, and watercress. (But be sure to steam or lightly cook, as when raw, many of these vegetables are goitrogens.) You may also need to use an iron supplement to get the ferritin levels up.

Reduce Exposure to Toxins

There are a variety of toxins out there in the environment that can affect the thyroid, and unfortunately we're exposed to them daily in our air, food, and water. Here are some of the specific toxins to keep in mind.

- Fluoride—In the past, fluoride was used as a treatment for hyperthyroidism. In large enough quantities, it can slow down the thyroid gland. If you want to avoid fluoride, the best thing is to avoid ingesting it. Drink water that is not fluoridated—a reverse osmosis filter can remove fluoride. And if you or your children need fluoride for your teeth, stick to topical forms, like toothpastes and rinses.

- Perchlorate—a by-product of rocket fuel and explosives manufacturing. It gets into the water supply and then into the food supply through the produce irrigated by that water. There's not much you can do to avoid eating perchlorate-contaminated foods, except to grow your own produce and water it with water that you've had tested for perchlorate contamination. If you drink well water, you should also have that water tested, and if you live in an area near a current or former production facility for rockets, explosives, or fireworks, consider having your water independently tested. And stay up on the latest news about perchlorate legislation—http://www.perchlorate.org is a great source of information.

- Perfluorooctanoic acid (PFOA) is an ingredient in many nonstick coatings on pans, stain-resistant and water-resistant coatings on carpets and fabrics, and in microwave popcorn bags—all things that you'll want to avoid. Look for PFOA-free labels and certifications on these kinds of products.

- Triclosan is found in some antibacterial soaps, hand sanitizers, and toiletries. It can also impair thyroid function, so you may want to avoid products that include this ingredient.

- Bisphenol-A—Abbreviated as BPA, bisphenol-A is used in a variety of plastic products. We're now seeing "BPA-free" labels on clear plastic water bottles and baby bottles. But you'll want to make sure that plastic food containers are also BPA free, and never microwave anything in a plastic container unless you're certain it's free of BPA.

- Mercury—We are exposed to mercury through dental fillings, and some fish—like tuna—have high levels of mercury. (Uh-oh, there go those sushi dates with Janell!) Mercury levels can be tested using hair analysis or blood tests. If you have excessive levels of mercury, you'll want to work with a practitioner who has expertise in the detoxification of heavy metals.

- Radiation—Be careful about unnecessary radiation exposure for you and your children. That means insisting that your dentist use a "thyroid collar," a lead collar placed around your neck, during dental X-rays. And beware of the routine annual dental X-rays—there should be a specific dental reason why they need to take dental X-rays—not just the "we need a new X-ray every year" excuse.

Dr. Christianson focuses on helping identify and remove toxins as part of his overall treatment approach to Hashimoto's and hypothyroidism. In my case, I had higher blood levels of both mercury and arsenic—and I had low copper and chromium levels—so he used supplements to perform a gentle detoxification.

According to Dr. Christianson:

When arsenic accumulates, it's usually from well water and tap water. The Scottsdale area has fairly high levels of arsenic in the water. You also find arsenic in treated furniture products and hardwoods from South and Central America. I had one couple as patients who had extremely high arsenic levels, and doctors even thought the husband had cancer. It turned out that the couple had just installed a custom kitchen, and the hardwoods were outgassing arsenic. Once they detoxed, their arsenic levels returned to normal and his symptoms disappeared.

MANAGE YOUR THYROID DURING PREGNANCY

In my case, I had a fairly easy first pregnancy with Spencer—minimal morning sickness, some fatigue but generally good energy—but that was before my thyroid diagnosis.

I still hadn't been diagnosed when I was pregnant with Hudson, but I now suspect it was already a problem, as I had more puffiness and bloating, I gained weight much more easily, and tried to be active but felt more tired than usual. One of the most noticeable symptoms for me was how puffy I was around the eyes—which I later learned can be a hypothyroidism symptom.

I'm pretty certain my thyroid was the culprit when, after Hudson, I was working with a trainer, working out several hours per day, and eating well, yet not much was happening in terms of weight loss. That's when I was at my most puffy and bloated, and my hair was brittle and broken—it looked like a lighter had singed it. My hair got so bad that Cale even had a water softener put in the house. We thought it was the water!

And then it turns out that the life-threatening atrial fibrillation in my pregnancy with Stella may also be linked to my Hashimoto's thyroiditis. I wish I had known more about the thyroid back when I was pregnant with Hudson, because pregnancy is often when thyroid problems first appear in some women.

For other women who already have a thyroid condition, pregnancy can be a time when symptoms calm down, but then they come roaring back to life after delivery, when the immune system kicks back into high gear. It can also be complicated to manage a thyroid condition during pregnancy, especially as many obstetricians don't know much about thyroid disease, and many endocrinologists don't know about pregnancy!

Here are some of the most important things to keep in mind about pregnancy and thyroid disease.

Hypothyroidism in a pregnant woman or unborn baby can have negative effects on the health of both. If a woman is hypothyroid before becoming pregnant, doctors recommend that her dosage be adjusted so that TSH is below 2.5 mIU/L prior to conception. This lowers the risk of the TSH going up during the first trimester of pregnancy. By the time a woman is four to six weeks pregnant, her dose of thyroid medication will usually need to be increased, potentially by as much as 50 percent. Some doctors suggest that a woman start taking a predetermined extra amount of medication the moment a pregnancy is confirmed (for example, even as early as a week post-conception, using a pregnancy test.) Thyroid testing should be done on a regular basis throughout pregnancy, especially during the first trimester.

If a woman is diagnosed as hypothyroid during pregnancy, she should be treated immediately, and the goal should be to rapidly restore her thyroid levels to normal. Doctors recommend that during the first trimester, the TSH level should be maintained at a level between 0.1 and 2.5 mIU/L; then 0.2 to 3.0 mIU/L during the second trimester, and 0.3 to 3.0 mIU/L in the third trimester.

A woman with Hashimoto's antibodies who has normal TSH levels in the early stages of her pregnancy is still at increased risk of becoming hypothyroid at some point during the pregnancy and should be monitored regularly through the pregnancy for elevated TSH.

If lower-than-normal TSH levels are detected in a pregnant woman, she should be evaluated to determine if the cause of her hyperthyroidism is transient hyperthyroidism/hyperemesis gravidarum—a condition of pregnancy that causes severe morning sickness—or Graves' disease. The diagnosis is made by determining if a woman has a goiter and/or tests positive for thyroid antibodies.

If you have active Graves' disease or hyperthyroidism, most doctors will suggest that you wait to get pregnant until your Graves'/hyperthyroidism is in remission or you've done something to permanently resolve the issue—i.e., surgery or radioactive iodine (RAI)—and are stabilized on a dosage of thyroid hormone replacement medication.

If a pregnant woman is hyperthyroid due to Graves' disease or nodules, the woman should begin hyperthyroidism treatment right away. Typically, pregnant women receive antithyroid drug treatment or, if a woman is an existing patient, her dosage will be adjusted so that free T4 levels remain in the normal range for someone who is not pregnant.

The antithyroid drug of choice (especially during the first trimester) is propylthiouracil, because methimazole has a slightly higher (though very small) risk of birth defects. Women are typically switched to methimazole for the second and third trimesters.

If a woman has a negative reaction to antithyroid drugs, requires very high doses to control her hyperthyroidism, or has uncontrolled hyperthyroidism despite treatment, surgery may be recommended, but only in the second trimester, when it poses the least risk. Radioactive iodine is not given to any woman who is or who might be pregnant.

If a new mother has Graves' disease, her newborn should be evaluated for thyroid dysfunction.

Breast-feeding is safe for a woman taking appropriate doses of thyroid hormone replacement drugs. For a nursing mother on antithyroid drugs, doctors recommend that the dosages be divided throughout the day, and taken at times after breast-feeding. Breast-feeding infants whose mothers are taking antithyroid drugs should have periodic thyroid function test screening.

Though universal thyroid screening in pregnant women is not currently a standard practice, screening and evaluation should take place among women who are at a higher risk of thyroid disease, including women:

with a personal history of thyroid dysfunction and/or thyroid surgery

with a family history of thyroid disease

with a goiter

with thyroid antibodies

with symptoms or clinical signs that may suggest hypothyroidism

with type 1 diabetes

with a history of either miscarriage or preterm delivery

with other autoimmune disorders that are often linked to autoimmune thyroid problems, such as vitiligo, adrenal

insufficiency, hypoparathyroidism, atrophic gastritis,
pernicious anemia, systemic sclerosis, systemic lupus
erythematosus, and Sjögren's syndrome

with infertility

who have previously received radiation to the head or neck
area as a cancer treatment, or who have had multiple dental
X-rays

who are morbidly obese, which is defined as a body mass index
(BMI) of over 40, or a body weight that is 20 percent or
more over ideal body weight

who are age thirty or older

who have been treated with amiodarone (Cordarone) for heart
rhythm irregularities

who have been treated with lithium

who, in the previous six weeks, have been exposed to iodine in
a medical test contrast agent

My advice for thyroid patients during pregnancy is to really
learn about pregnancy and your hormones, get to know your
body, and to pay attention to signs and symptoms. My mom gave
me good advice on a down day—she said, "This is only tempo-
rary, and before you know it, you'll be saying the same thing to
your daughter." It's true! Remind yourself that your body is mor-
phing into a superhero baby-making machine, and that it's really
a short time and goes by faster than you realize, so embrace it, and
enjoy it if you can. I think that the most useful thing for me was
keeping physically active—it doesn't have to be rigorous, but I
liked yoga and swimming—as it really helped me feel less creaky
and improved my mood.

Ursula explains her ups and downs through pregnancy:

After I gave birth to my first child, a beautiful baby boy, I loved being a mom, but I felt anxious and run-down, like I was in a daze. I had insomnia and sometimes didn't sleep for nights in a row, my heart rate at rest was spiking to 170 beats per minute, I would pass out in the shower due to the heat of the water, my hair fell out in clumps, and people thought I had an eating disorder. But I dismissed everything because I thought it was because I was a new mom. I was put on antianxiety medications—then, about a year later, I was having some vision problems, and noticed one of my eyes was swollen. Only then did my doctor do bloodwork. I remember hearing my doctor tell me I had thyroid eye disease and Graves' disease. A big weight fell off my shoulders . . . at least there was a name for how I had been feeling, and I was finally on the road to recovery. I was put on propanolol, PTU and prednisone. I put on thirty pounds in six weeks—and it left my eyes unchanged. I was advised not to become pregnant again, but a few months later, I was expecting my second child. I ended up going into remission—and went on to have a third child, and since then my levels have stayed the same since.

Marissa shares her story:

When I was pregnant with my oldest son, I went from 115 pounds to 215 in nine months. I blamed it on eating horribly and not exercising. I was miserable. I had NEVER been heavy in my life. I was able to get most of the weight off by the time my son was two, but I couldn't understand why I was so tired, my hair was falling out, my skin was dry. I was trying to get pregnant again, but couldn't. I went to the doctor, only to have them tell me I was depressed. They tried to give me antide-pressant medication, and I refused. I went to another doctor who did some tests and found out my thyroid was pretty much nonfunctioning.

It can be challenging to find the right doctors, tests, and treatments, and it frequently is a trial-and-error process, but believe me, it's worth it. When you finally wake up one day feeling energetic, and like yourself again, it's the best feeling in the world.

6

Hormone Balance: The Three-Legged Stool

Health is the greatest possession.

—LAO TZU

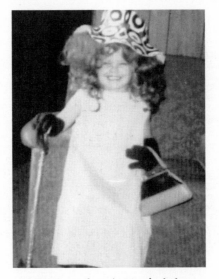

Gena, age three, in Mom's clothes and ultracool 1970s wig and hat

We've delved into the thyroid, but it's important to look at how the thyroid fits into the overall hormone balance, and the challenges of achieving and maintaining that balance. Mary and I both like the example created by Drs. Richard and Karilee Shames, who are authors of a number of terrific books on thyroid and hormonal health (listed in the Resources section). They refer to our hormone balance as a three-legged stool.

One leg of the stool is our reproductive hormones, specifically the female hormones, for us women. That's mainly the estrogens and progesterone, and they go up and down, depending where you are in your menstrual cycle. Levels of these hormones get particularly high during pregnancy, and they crash back down to the normal—or even low—levels after pregnancy. From your first period until you hit menopause, these hormones typically cycle every month. The first half of your cycle, from when you get your period, until when you ovulate, things are usually fairly calm. But then, as progesterone and estrogen rise during the second half of the cycle, that's when PMS symptoms can show up, and you can feel more tired and draggy. We women also have some testosterone, though it is of course associated more with men. Testosterone helps us to build and maintain muscle, and it also contributes to a healthy sex drive.

The next leg of the stool is our adrenal hormones. The adrenals are tiny glands, shaped like peanuts, and they sit over the kidneys. They produce the hormones that help our body cope with stress, whether it's physical stress like a poor diet or ongoing infection, chronic stress like not getting enough sleep or a traffic-filled daily commute, or major life stressors like a breakup, losing a job, or a death in the family. If you're bombarded by stress on a regular basis, the adrenals can sometimes become less effective, and you end up with what's called adrenal fatigue or adrenal insufficiency. You can also feel tired, and you may find it hard to exercise. You may also notice that you easily catch every infection going around, and that it takes longer to recuperate.

The third leg of the stool is, you guessed it, the thyroid.

We've talked quite a bit about the thyroid, but the key thing to remember is that your thyroid gland is responsible for producing the hormones that deliver oxygen and energy to *each and every cell, organ, tissue, and gland in the body.* That's a huge job. And when it's not working properly, it's a disaster, because that oxygen and energy doesn't get to where it needs to be—your brain, your heart, your bloodstream, your digestive system—even your hair and nails.

The balanced stool metaphor is important because any imbalance in one leg of the stool means that you can't be balanced, and the stool tips over. So, when reproductive hormones drop significantly, as they do after age forty, or chronic stress is just whipping you, or your thyroid has gone south, it's almost impossible to have hormonal balance in all three legs of your stool.

For example, it's difficult for the thyroid to work properly if the adrenals aren't in good shape. And if your adrenals aren't working well, the body tends to slow down on reproductive hormone production. And if the thyroid isn't doing what it's supposed to, nothing else is getting the energy it needs to function properly.

The key is balance: balance in each area, and balance among the different hormones. Here are some of the things I've learned that may help you in your own journey to wellness.

KEEP TRACK OF YOUR REPRODUCTIVE/ SEX HORMONES

Many times, we don't really think to check our hormone levels until we're well into perimenopause, or we're having trouble getting pregnant, or our sex drive has gone kaput. Whether you're in your twenties or over forty, reproductive and precursor hormones are important to understand and monitor.

In my case, in my early forties, I'm paying attention to the fact that the fluctuations in, and over time the decline of, estrogen and progesterone levels have already started. It's typical for that to begin when you hit your late thirties. Those fluctuations may also be a trigger for, or coincide with, thyroid slowdown. I can't tell you how many of my girlfriends in their early forties and beyond are now starting to get diagnosed with thyroid issues!

But at any point along the way, it's a really good idea to get a baseline idea of where these hormones are.

If you are already dealing with thyroid issues, it can be very useful to take a look at these reproductive hormones. Adding in progesterone can sometimes be the difference between a thyroid treatment that works and one that falls flat. And in some cases, if you're estrogen dominant—where the estrogen/progesterone ratio is imbalanced—you may find yourself with weight gain and bloating that no amount of thyroid treatment can resolve.

The key is to work with a practitioner who has expertise in hormones. Again, these are usually the integrative physicians, naturopaths, bioidentical hormone experts, and some of the great gynecologists who focus on hormonal balance.

There is so much more involved in the whole hormone issue that I can't get into here. But if you want to really delve in more deeply, I recommend Mary Shomon's book *The Thyroid Hormone Breakthrough* (if you're not yet in perimenopause, or you're trying to get pregnant, are pregnant, or breast-feeding) or her book *The Menopause Thyroid Solution* (if you're over forty and want to balance your hormones).

Tips for a Better Sex Drive

Part of being Thyroid Sexy is, well, having sex, right?! But when you're hypothyroid, let's face it, sometimes you are so not in the mood.

One study found that as many as 43 percent of women have some sort of sexual dysfunction, including low desire, and/or pain during intercourse. And if you polled thyroid patients, the number would be higher, because low sex drive is a common—but not often talked about—symptom of hypothyroidism. Plus, it's much more common in women over forty. Uh-oh!

If you suffer from low sex drive, first you need to be sure that you are getting optimal thyroid treatment—including testing your TSH, T4/T3 levels, and seeing if there's a need for additional T3 or natural thyroid. Also make sure that your estrogen, progesterone, and testosterone are checked. You may benefit from some hormone treatment—and in particular, prescription testosterone—that can help with libido.

Keep in mind that other prescription drugs such as antidepressants, tranquilizers, and antihypertensives—as well as many illegal drugs such as cocaine and marijuana—can reduce your sex drive.

Make sure you exercise. It improves blood flow and helps increase desire, triggers greater sexual confidence and frequency, and enhances the ability to be aroused and achieve orgasm—no matter what your age! Sounds good to us!

Lose weight. Even ten to twenty pounds can allow estrogen and testosterone to return to proper balance, and boost your confidence on top of it all!

Try therapy or couples counseling. If relationship issues are getting in the way, your sex life may be the first place to show it. A few sessions with a good couples counselor or sex therapist can work wonders.

Talk to your health professional about over-the-counter supplements that may help with sex drive, including arginine, Asian ginseng (panax), avena-sativa/oat extract, damiana, horny goat weed (yes, that's really the name!), and Royal Maca (a special formulation of maca from Whole World Botanicals; see page 162).

Thyroid patients in our communities have also had great ideas about how to stay sexy and feel sexy . . .

"A hot, luxurious bubble bath works every time!"—Lori

"Take a hot shower, wash my hair, put on makeup and some perfume, a nice outfit or lingerie, and remember why I love my husband so much!"—Helen

"I go to the gym and work out. Releasing that stress at the gym helps me feel much sexier and better."—Ana

"I am extremely blessed to have a husband who even on my worst days tells me I look beautiful! I pick myself back up, do my hair and makeup, and away I go."—Kristen

BE PREPARED FOR PERIMENOPAUSE

It's so important to be prepared for perimenopause.

Did you know that perimenopause can begin as early as your thirties? I know—just the word *menopause* sounds, so, well, old. I'm not ready to star in the remake of *Golden Girls*!

But perimenopause is not the same as menopause. Menopause is when your period has already stopped for a year—usually around age fifty or shortly after. But the fluctuating hormones of perimenopause can go on for a decade or more before periods finally stop. So if you, like me, are in your forties, you're in perimenopause!

I've decided that I'm going to embrace it! Being an empowered, educated patient and having my life experience and some hard knocks—these are the very things that make me stronger . . . and sexier! Menopause is the next step of life . . . so bring it on!

This time of life can be particularly confusing for women, though, because thyroid problems often show up at the same age as perimenopausal or menopausal symptoms, and they share many of the same symptoms. Actually, except for traditional hot flashes and night sweats that last a few minutes, vaginal/bladder problems, and sagging/tender breasts, the rest of the symptoms of perimenopause and menopause are usually the same as the symptoms of a thyroid problem. If you're experiencing any of these symptoms and are assuming that it's perimenopause or menopause, think again, and make sure you also have your thyroid checked or rechecked.

It's also a time when, even if you've gotten your thyroid under control and you're cruising along, the ups and downs of perimenopause can start to destabilize your thyroid. There are a variety of ways to help protect yourself and make the whole process easier.

Mary Shomon's *The Menopause Thyroid Solution* explains it all in detail. (She never did like that title, though. She says that she's always wished it were called *Hormone Balance After 40*. And admittedly, it'd be much easier to be seen carrying it around!) It's a good read, and will help you understand all the hormonal shifts—thyroid, reproductive hormones, and adrenals—that go on after forty.

There's no definitive test for perimenopause, but usually, doctor will look for changes in the menstrual period, and the most common symptoms, like hot flashes and night sweats. A gynecologist can also, in a pelvic exam, see changes to the outer layer of the vagina and changes to the uterus and ovaries that take place as you get closer to menopause. There's no official "perimenopause blood test," but they can check hormones like follicle-stimulating hormone (FSH) and luteinizing hormone (LH)—they tend to go up as you get closer to menopause, though they can fluctuate quite a bit until then. You can also check the different types of estrogen—estradiol, estrone, and estriol. Reductions in estradiol, and increases in estrone and estriol, are more common as you get closer to menopause.

Remember, if you have a doctor or HMO that just won't run these tests, you can get them yourself with a patient-directed laboratory service like MyMedLab or with saliva hormone test kits.

Here are some things that I'm going to keep in mind as I go through perimenopause, and later, menopause, myself:

- Have a great relationship with your doctor. (And if you don't have that doctor in your life, make it a point to find him or her.)

- Listen to your body—trust and know when something doesn't feel right. I sometimes joke around and call it my Spidey sense, but if you really tune in, you'll be much more on top of things.
- Get regular checkups, along with recommended Pap smears, mammograms, bone density checks, and other screening tests.
- Make sure to have baseline sex hormones checked before things start to shift too much, and then periodically monitor them to keep track of whether they're in balance.

MONITORING AND SUPPLEMENTING WITH HORMONES

There are some important hormones to check—and to supplement if necessary. (But remember—hormones are not like vitamins—even if they're available over-the-counter, you should always have a doctor's oversight when supplementing with hormones.)

According to David Borenstein, an integrative physician in Manhattan, it's important to consider the reproductive hormones and how they interact with the adrenals and the thyroid.

In particular, I'm often looking at the progesterone levels. In women with low progesterone, supplementing with progesterone can often provide tremendous benefits. I also look for estrogen dominance—whether due to low estrogen with very low progesterone, or high estrogen versus lower progesterone. Again, addressing the adrenals and supplementing with progesterone are often crucial to restoring balance in the overall hormonal system. There's also a concept called the "cortisol steal," where chronic stress means that the body decreases production of the sex hormones and aldosterone. Helping the adrenals can help prevent this. When appropriate, I also prescribe bioidentical hormones as needed.

Pregnenolone

Pregnenolone is a precursor hormone to reproductive and adrenal hormones. Levels can be checked and imbalances detected with blood tests. Many practitioners recommend keeping doses below 5 to 10 mg a day, because too much can cause palpitations, acne, irritability, hair loss, insomnia, and headaches.

Dehydroepiandrosterone (DHEA)

DHEA is a precursor to reproductive and adrenal hormones. It's available over-the-counter, but you should stick to prescription or a pharmaceutical-grade brand. (One recommended by many doctors we know is the DHEA from Enzymatic Therapies.) Again, many doctors have told us that women should probably not be taking more than 5 to 10 mg a day as too much DHEA can cause acne, growth of facial hair in women, deepening voice, irritability, hair loss, menstrual irregularities, sleep disruptions, and other symptoms we definitely do not want!

Progesterone

Progesterone is a key reproductive hormone. Progesterone replacement drugs—known as progestogens—include synthetic progesterone analogues (called progestins) and natural, bioidentical progesterone. Many of the integrative doctors we know recommend that women avoid the synthetic progestins, because of their association with an increased risk of stroke and breast cancer, as well as menstrual irregularities, weight gain, drowsiness, depression, fatigue, and a long list of other symptoms. Some holistic doctors believe that bioidentical progesterone carries far less risk, and that for thyroid patients, progesterone may help the body better use thyroid hormone and counteract estrogen dominance

Synthetic progestins are found in a number of brands of progestogen drugs—their generic names are medroxyprogesterone/MPA, norethindrone, norethindrone acetate, norgestrel, and megestrol acetate. You also want to be aware that the synthetic progestin levonorgestrel is used in hormonal IUDs, that there are synthetic progestin-only birth control pills (called the "mini pill"), and that progestin is delivered via implants and injections for birth control.

Typically, hormone experts and integrative physicians recommend bioidentical progesterone, which is available in several manufactured forms, including Prometrium—an oral capsule (it uses peanut oil as its suspension, in case you have allergies), and various vaginal progesterone gels such as Prochieve and Crinone. Bioidentical progesterone is also available from compounding pharmacies in various forms, including capsules, transdermal creams, vaginal creams, vaginal suppositories, sublingual pills and drops, troches (lozenges dissolved between cheek and gum), and implantable pellets.

There are also lower-dose progesterone creams available over-the-counter. Keep in mind that many of them do not have consistent or guaranteed amounts of progesterone in them. But some brands that doctors we know regularly recommend are ProGest

Cream from Emerita and Kevala's PureGest. Again, make sure the doctor is guiding you on how much to use and how to use it.

Testosterone

In women, testosterone is often checked if there is low—or no—sex drive. Some doctors will recommend low-dose testosterone supplements for women to help with sexual desire, energy, and muscle building in women. The only forms of supplemental testosterone typically used for women are gels and pellets. Compounding pharmacies can do capsules, but many practitioners prefer that women not take testosterone orally.

Testosterone is available only by prescription, so you'll need a doctor's direction. Keep in mind that it needs to be used with care, as it can cause acne, hair loss, growth of facial hair in women, oilier skin, a deepening of the voice, and a reduction in good cholesterol and an increase in bad cholesterol.

Estrogens

Estrogen is a reproductive hormone that has an impact on thyroid function—positive and negative—affects fertility, and has an impact on a variety of health issues throughout a woman's life.

Dr. Kevin Passero, a Washington, D.C.–based naturopathic physician, explains why estrogen balance in particular is crucial for thyroid patients:

> Sex hormones, particularly estrogen, play an important role in thyroid hormone balance and thyroid function. It is a well-known fact that thyroid function can change drastically during pregnancy due to estrogen surges. This interplay between the

hormones can play out in a more subtle but equally important fashion when sex hormone imbalances exist. Properly testing and assessing sex hormones is a critical part of managing thyroid disorders.

Estrogen can be tested with laboratory blood tests, blood spot testing, and with saliva hormone testing, to evaluate levels and assess imbalances.

With estrogen, like progesterone, the conventional approach to supplementing focuses on one category of estrogen—in this case, conjugated estrogens—which are typically mixtures of a variety of estrogens from horses. Most integrative and holistic hormone experts we've consulted advise against use of conjugated estrogen drugs—in oral, cream, suppository, or patch form—as they are most often associated with the negative side effects of estrogen therapy.

Integrative physicians typically recommend 17-Beta Estradiol (17ß-estradiol), also known as "bioidentical estrogen." It comes in oral pills, as well as transdermal gel/cream/lotion/mist/patch, vaginal cream, vaginal ring, and vaginal tablet forms. Compounding pharmacies offer a variety of forms of estrogen, including "Bi-est," which mixes bioidentical estriol and 17ß-estradiol, and "Tri-est," which is a mixture of bioidentical versions of all three key estrogens: estriol, estrone, and 17ß-estradiol.

If you need estrogen, and you still have a uterus, remember that your doctor will need to prescribe an accompanying progestogen to "oppose" the estrogen and prevent buildup of your endometrial lining.

Many women get through perimenopause without needing any sort of estrogen therapy, but if you are really struggling with the symptoms that respond best to estrogen—like hot flashes, night sweats, vaginal dryness or atrophy, and recurrent urinary infections—and your doctor recommends prescription treatment, consider using the lowest effective dose of medication, for the shortest time necessary to relieve symptoms, and in a transdermal, bioidentical form when possible, to minimize risks and side effects.

Keep in mind that conventional medicine says you should never take estrogen therapy if you:

have undiagnosed or abnormal genital bleeding

currently have breast cancer, or have a suspicious lump

have a suspected or confirmed estrogen-dependent benign or
cancerous tumor or growth

have any history of clots in the legs (deep vein thrombosis,
DVT) or lungs (pulmonary embolism)

have had a stroke or a heart attack in the past year, or in some
cases, at some point in the past

have any liver dysfunction

Estrogen is also strongly discouraged by conventional physicians if you:

have a family history of blood clots, strokes, heart disease,
breast disease, or cancer

have migraine headaches

have gallbladder disease

smoke cigarettes

TAKE CARE OF YOUR ADRENALS

I want to talk about the adrenal glands, because adrenal health is so important to thyroid health, and it's definitely been an issue for me, and a factor that has contributed to my fatigue.

As I mentioned earlier, the adrenal glands produce our stress hormones. One of the key hormones is cortisol, which is released as part of the daily hormonal cycle. Then there's adrenaline, which is typically released when your body decides that you're in a really stressful crisis situation. Adrenaline is released as a fight-or-flight response, going back to the days when we humans needed to run away from wild animals. (I did some of that on the *Sheena* set!)

Cortisol helps your body become more effective at producing glucose from proteins and is designed to increase the body's energy in times of stress. Adrenaline makes you energetic and alert and quickly increases metabolism. It also helps fat cells release energy. As the adrenal hormones go up and down in response to various stressors, they help balance blood sugar.

But these days, that fight-or-flight response often kicks in all the time, whether you're sitting in a traffic jam, having an argument, trying to get the kids to school, or worrying about a project at work—or working ninety-hour weeks, not eating well, and living on too little sleep, like I did. Being consistently under stress takes a toll on the adrenal glands, and eventually they can run out of steam and stop producing sufficient hormones. You end up feeling "tired but wired."

Dr. Kevin Passero, a naturopathic physician, explains why adrenal health is so important to thyroid treatment:

There is no other system related to thyroid health that is more overlooked than the adrenal glands. These small glands located above the kidneys are responsible for managing all stress in your body. What most people don't understand is that thyroid hormone in its own way is a stress on the body. Take, for example, a person who has been prescribed a slight overdose of thyroid medicine. They feel anxious and jittery, have trouble sleeping and often experience heart racing . . . all symptoms related to stress. The point is that if the adrenal system is not strong, the thyroid will automatically alter its function to accommodate a weaker resilience to stress. I have seen many people with borderline thyroid issues have those issues fully resolved just by doing appropriate therapy with the adrenal system. In the majority of the other thyroid cases, I see the adrenal system plays an equally important role, even though the thyroid needs to be addressed directly. The interplay of adrenal hormones, particularly cortisol, and thyroid hormones is so closely related it is a huge disservice to not take both into account. Properly testing and assessing adrenal hormones is a critical part of managing thyroid disorders.

What sorts of signs might indicate that you have adrenal fatigue?

Excessive fatigue and exhaustion
Sleeping seven or eight hours yet wake up exhausted
Continuing to wake up in the middle of the night, and
    sometimes not being able to go back to sleep
Feeling overwhelmed by or unable to cope with stressors

Feeling run-down

Craving salty and sweet foods

Feeling most energetic in the evening

Experiencing low stamina, slow to recover from exercise

Being slow to recover from injury, illness, time changes, or jet
   lag

Having difficulty concentrating, brain fog

Poor digestion

Low immune function

Worsening food or environmental allergies

Premenstrual syndrome or difficulties that develop during
   menopause

Consistent low blood pressure

Extreme sensitivity to cold

Excess mood responses after eating carbohydrates

Dark circles under the eyes

Momentary lightheadedness after standing up

Cystic breasts

A history of mononucleosis and/or Epstein Barr virus
   reactivation

Conventional endocrinologists and conventional tests don't diagnose adrenal fatigue, because they are prepared to diagnose only major diseases, not imbalances, in the adrenals. An integrative, holistic, or complementary practitioner is more prepared to evaluate symptoms and signs of milder or more subtle adrenal dysfunction, using the 24-hour saliva cortisol and DHEA tests. You can get these test kits from your doctors, and they are also available as self-tests.

If evidence of adrenal imbalance or fatigue is found, some

integrative physicians and naturopaths recommend adaptogenic supplements, such as ashwaganda. Adaptogens are supplements that help restore balance to systems in the body, whether an increase or decrease is needed. There are also a variety of other herbs, vitamins, and glandulars that may help support and heal the adrenal glands. In some cases where adrenal insufficiency may be more severe, some integrative physicians prescribe low doses of hydrocortisone, a bioidentical form of the hormone cortisol.

Sara Gottfried, MD, author of *The Hormone Cure*, sees a lot of adrenal fatigue in her practice, and she often recommends that the key first steps toward relief are to begin stress-reducing practices, make dietary changes, and add some supplements.

> Even eight minutes of meditation or a fifteen-minute yoga practice can help modulate cortisol. Protein, especially at breakfast, also is increasingly important when the adrenals are out of balance. Starbucks and a muffin is not an acceptable breakfast. I also find that most people will feel better if I start them on supplements such as B vitamins, vitamin C, B_5 pantothenic acid, and in some cases, the adaptogenic herbs.

New York City–based holistic physician David Borenstein, MD, explains his approach to adrenal health:

> I think it's extremely important to address adrenal function as a foundation before attempting to balance other hormones. I'm a big believer in addressing adrenals concurrently or before thyroid replacement. To evaluate the adrenals, I typically run a four-point saliva cortisol and DHEA-S, and I also use blood tests to evaluate morning cortisol, aldosterone, and ACTH.

To treat adrenal imbalances, I often use nutritional supplements along with dietary recommendations, stress reduction, exercise modification, and a focus on improving sleep. Supplements I have recommended for adrenal support include adrenal glandulars, vitamin C, licorice, ginseng, and ashwaganda, among others. If patients have high cortisol at night, I often recommend phosphatidyl serine, l-theanine, and calming herbs. Nutritionally, I counsel patients to follow a low-glycemic diet, avoiding sugar, coffee, and other stimulants. When medication is needed, I prescribe the minimum amount of low-dose hydrocortisone (Cortef), with the goal of short-term, judicious use so as to allow other factors to help restore adrenal balance.

Making sure you get enough sleep is also very important for the adrenals. Sleep is the time when adrenal hormones are restored and levels are rebalanced. When you're short on sleep, you're shortchanging your adrenals, lowering your immune system, and making it harder to lose weight to boot. (Not to mention, you're going to be even more tired than you need to be!)

Do keep in mind that many traditional endocrinologists don't acknowledge the existence of adrenal fatigue, adrenal insufficiency, or "adrenal burnout." They are about a decade or more behind the integrative physicians. (It's similar to the situation we saw a decade ago, when integrative physicians recognized "prediabetes" and insulin resistance, while endocrinologists only acknowledged that there was a cutoff point at which diabetes should be diagnosed.)

Getting Good-Quality Sleep

You may be spending eight or more hours in bed, but are you getting enough good-quality sleep? Many new smartphone apps and devices can evaluate how much restorative sleep you're getting, how many times you awake, and the quality of the sleep. You can also set up a video camera to tape yourself, or ask a partner or family member to do an informal "sleep study," to see if you are snoring or having episodes of sleep apnea where you briefly stop breathing. (This is more common in thyroid patients.) If any of these behaviors are observed, you should definitely have a formal, medically supervised sleep study.

If you can't sleep, here are some tips:

- Don't work in bed.
- Don't watch television or read in bed.
- Minimize light in your bedroom.
- Limit naps.
- Avoid stimulants before bed.
- Keep your bedroom cool.
- Take a cool shower or bath before bed.
- Add a light protein and carbohydrate bedtime snack before bed.
- Try a nonprescription sleep aid like diphenylhydramine (Benadryl, Tylenol PM, Excedrin PM) or Doxylamine (Unisom For Sleep).
- Try a low dose of melatonin, an over-the-counter hormone, as a sleep aid.
- Take a magnesium/calcium supplement at bedtime.

- Talk to your doctor about prescription sleep medications, such as zolpidem (Ambien), triazolam (Halcion), temazepam (Restoril), zaleplon (Sonata), or eszopiclone (Lunesta).
- Talk to the doctor about antidepressants, antianxiety drugs, and muscle relaxants, which are sometimes prescribed to help improve sleep.

A variety of herbs can be helpful for sleep, including valerian and hops. Valerian functions as a sedative and can help with quality of sleep and insomnia. Hops is thought to be more beneficial to help you stay asleep. One of our favorite doctors, Jacob Teitelbaum, MD, has combined them—as well as other sleep-promoting ingredients like l-theanine—in a supplement called Revitalizing Sleep Formula, from Enzymatic Therapies. A great book that talks about approaches to getting high-quality, restorative sleep is Dr. Teitelbaum's *From Fatigued to Fantastic*.

Is It Perimenopause or Thyroid?

It can be confusing to women—and their doctors—whether symptoms that show up in our forties are symptoms of a new (or existing) thyroid condition or signs of perimenopause—the period prior to menopause when reproductive hormone levels start to fluctuate.

Here are some of the common perimenopause symptoms that can also be thyroid symptoms:

- Irregular menstrual cycle, spotting
- Heavier periods
- Sleep problems/insomnia/frequent waking
- Weight gain/redistribution of weight to belly and waist
- Mood changes
- Lower sex drive/loss of sex drive
- Hair loss
- Itchiness/tingling in the skin, extremities
- Reduced bone density
- Elevated cholesterol levels
- Fatigue, lack of energy
- Body aches and pains
- Brain fog; difficulty concentrating and with memory
- Changes in chronic headaches/migraines

Symptoms that are more common to perimenopause than thyroid disease:

- Hot flashes/night sweats
- Change in PMS symptoms
- Vaginal dryness
- More frequent bladder infections
- Loss of skin elasticity, wrinkles

MARY SHOMON'S "M&M" MENOPAUSE SOLUTIONS

Mary, who is almost ten years to the day older than me, has already laid the groundwork for me to go through perimenopause better informed and prepared, since I have read *The Menopause Thyroid Solution.*

Mary really stayed on top of keeping her thyroid in balance, but in the course of going through perimenopause, she did not want to take prescription hormones—her mother had a hormone-sensitive breast cancer, so Mary and her doctor really wanted to avoid estrogen for menopausal symptoms.

Mary relied on two natural supplements that helped her quite a bit. She calls it the "M&M solution"—no, sorry—not the chocolates! It's Royal Maca and melatonin.

Mary started taking Royal Maca—a particular formulation of organic maca from a company called Whole World Botanicals. The Royal Maca is cooked, unlike most of the maca on the market, which is raw, goitrogenic, and not recommended for thyroid patients.

Maca has traditionally been used for centuries by the native people of the Andes in South America for fertility, sex drive, and PMS and menopause symptoms. It does not contain estrogen, but is adaptogenic—it helps the hormonal system achieve balance, up or down, as needed.

Within a few days of starting the Royal Maca, Mary's several-times-a-day hot flashes disappeared.

Maca also reportedly helps with thyroid function for people with Hashimoto's and hypothyroidism. According to the leading authority on maca in the United States, Whole World Botanicals' founder Dr. Viana Muller: "I was surprised to receive feedback from hundreds of women with hypothyroid issues who have benefited from taking Royal Maca. Most of them were having other hormonal imbalances, such as PMS, perimenopausal, or menopausal symptoms and discovered 'accidentally' how much better they felt when combining Royal Maca with their thyroid medication."

Mary discovered melatonin for menopause by accident.

Many women are aware of the benefits of melatonin as a sleep aid, but what you may not realize is that melatonin can have powerful hormonal effects for women in perimenopause and menopause.

Melatonin is a hormone produced by the pineal gland, a tiny gland located in the brain. The pineal is the master controller of our body's clock, including our day-to-day circadian clock that tells us when to sleep and when to wake, and the biological clock that decides on bigger hormonal issues, such as when we enter puberty and menopause.

The pineal gland controls the circadian rhythm—our daily cycle of sleeping and waking—by releasing a hormone called melatonin, produced primarily at night. Melatonin synthesis and release is stimulated by darkness.

The pineal also contains thyrotropin-releasing hormone (TRH), which the pineal uses to tell the pituitary to produce TSH. Melatonin is also apparently instrumental in the breakdown of T4 into T3, creating heat and energy.

Based on its role in circadian rhythm and sleep, melatonin has become well known as a helpful sleep aid, as a treatment to help prevent jet lag and reset the body clock to a new time zone, and for night-shift workers who have difficulty sleeping.

Mary started using it for sleep and noticed that she was waking up in the morning feeling more energetic and in a good mood. And even though she was smack dab in the middle of totally erratic periods—lasting two weeks, then not coming for three months, and so on—after two months on melatonin, her periods came back, and returned totally to normal . . . normal length, twenty-eight-day cycle, regular heaviness. She delved in to figure out what was going on and ended up connecting with Dr. Walter Pierpaoli, the world's top expert on melatonin and author of the bestseller *The Melatonin Miracle: Nature's Age-Reversing, Disease-Fighting, Sex-Enhancing Hormone.*

It turns out that helping with sleep is only one of many things that melatonin can do. According to Dr. Pierpaoli, it helps re-synch the body's daily sleep cycles, and the hormonal cycles— daily, monthly, and lifetime—as well!

Dr. Pierpaoli says that if we take a small dose of supplemental melatonin—he suggests no more than 3 mg of time-release melatonin nightly, an hour before bedtime, or by 11 p.m. but no later— the pineal gland can rest, and slow down the body's "expiration clock," so to speak.

(He's done studies that found that giving melatonin could even extend fertility in women in their forties, and return post-menopausal women in their late fifties to normal menstrual cycles!)

There's also evidence that melatonin increases estrogen levels, improves thyroid function, improves T4-to-T3 conversion, improves sensitivity to insulin, reduces blood sugar, and reduces luteinizing hormone and follicle-stimulating hormone in women under forty.

Dr. Pierpaoli calls melatonin the "queen of all hormones," which monitors and directs the whole "hormonal orchestra."

If you're interested in supplementing with melatonin, make sure to use only synthetic—not animal—melatonin. Dr. Pierpaoli formulated his own nonprescription, pharmaceutical-grade melatonin called TI-Melatonin, which many folks swear by.

Sometimes people worry about melatonin for autoimmune patients, but Dr. Pierpaoli and other experts say that this is a mistaken fear, and that melatonin is actually good for autoimmune patients. According to Dr. Pierpaoli, it helps restore normal immune reaction, and melatonin doesn't increase antibody production but instead helps address the underlying autoimmune imbalances.

COPING WITH FATIGUE

One of the most common symptoms of hormone imbalances—whether thyroid, sex hormones, or adrenals—is fatigue. Fatigue has always been one of the worst symptoms for me, as you know.

So I'm here to say, "Don't go through life tired."

The most important thing is, of course, to make sure that the thyroid treatment is optimized. For me, getting on a natural thyroid drug was key. But even then, I still find myself struggling at times to have enough energy to get through the day.

Ribose: A Great Supplement for Energy

In his terrific book *Beat Sugar Addiction Now*, Jacob Teitelbaum, MD—who works with thyroid, adrenal, chronic fatigue, and fibromyalgia patients—strongly recommends the supplement ribose to help with energy. Says Dr. Teitelbaum:

> When you are exhausted, your body craves sugar as it tries to get an energy boost. A special type of sugar called ribose is an excellent nutrient for energy production. In addition to its role in making DNA and RNA, ribose is

the key building block for generating energy. In fact, the main energy molecules in your body (ATP, FADH, etc.) are made of ribose plus B vitamins or phosphate. Ribose does not raise blood sugar or feed yeast overgrowth, yet it looks and tastes like sugar. Consequently, sugar addicts can use it as a sugar substitute. It actually has a negative value on the glycemic index. Ribose even tends to lower blood sugar in diabetics and may contribute to weight loss as well. Ribose will give you a powerful energy boost. Start with a 5,000 mg scoop of ribose three times a day for three to six weeks, then decrease to one scoop twice a day. If you get hyper from being too energized, lower the dose. Any brand of ribose is okay, as long as it is in powder form and you take the proper dose. Quality control problems have occurred outside of the United States, so buy a brand that uses "Bioenergy" ribose.

Here are some things that are really essential to feeling and looking good every day:

Get enough sleep. Again, it sounds so obvious, but with a houseful of children, and activities, and so much to do, it can be hard. Most of us need about seven or eight hours a night, religiously, to keep energy going, and to help hormones do their work. No fair complaining that you're tired if you are trying to get by on four or five hours a night.

Another thing that can affect your energy is a low dehydroepiandrosterone (DHEA) level. DHEA functions as part of both the reproductive and adrenal hormone systems. Have your

DHEA levels checked—your doctor can do this blood test, or you can order it yourself. If DHEA is low, it might be worth supplementing with a low dose of a good-quality DHEA, which you can get over the counter. (I like Enzymatic Therapy's pharmaceutical-grade DHEA, in 5 mg tablets.) Remember though, that taking DHEA is something you only do with your physician monitoring, because DHEA is still a hormone. (And too much can make your skin break out and cause you to sprout chin hairs, which are definitely not fun side effects.)

Make sure you're getting enough B vitamins, especially vitamin B_{12}, which is essential for energy. Consider taking a B complex plus B_{12} separately in a sublingual form (dissolves under the tongue) to make sure you're really absorbing it. Or you may even want to talk to the doctor about getting periodic B_{12} shots. I've done that at times, and it can really help energy.

Resist the temptation of those giant lattes, caffeine energy drinks, or other stimulants. They may rev you up for a little while but they're killers for your adrenal system. They make the adrenal glands work harder and can end up further exhausting them. Things to avoid include caffeine, ephedra, guarana, kola nut, and prescription stimulants. For energy, I like kombucha (fermented tea) drinks, like JT's, which you can get at Whole Foods and other health food stores. They're low in calories, but they give you a nice energy boost without the buzz of caffeine.

Coping Secrets from Thyroid Patients

We asked patients in our thyroid support communities to share their own tips about how they cope when they don't feel energetic enough to keep up with work, family, and household duties. Here are some of their thoughts:

"I remember that it's not selfish to take time for yourself. You can't fill other people's glasses if your own isn't full. I know it sounds clichéd, but it was a hard-learned lesson. My favorite thing is a bubble bath with a little wine and some music. It doesn't have to be for more than twenty minutes, but the quiet time to think or read does wonders for me."—Rae

"I drink coffee, and if that doesn't help, I just give in and take a nap. I have given up long ago on keeping the house perfectly clean. I try to get things done when I do have energy so that I don't beat myself up when I don't and I can't."—Tish

"I take vitamin B_{12} for energy. It helps me get my day moving."—Ann

"I try to have a swim. It reboots my energy. Water is a lovely healer. Other days I just push through and collapse into bed at the end of the day. As a teacher I have to create my own energy to deal with work some days, particularly in summer."—Lynette

Some patients have found that prioritizing and keeping busy is a help.

"I actually find that the more I have on my to-do list—I schedule lots of things—the less time I have time to think about being tired."—Jessica

"On days like that, I ask myself, 'what is the most important thing that needs to get done today?' Whatever the answer is, that is what I concentrate on. On really bad days, I make sure all needs are met, but I keep it super simple (pizza, anyone?). I have four kids—one of whom has multiple therapy appointments a week—and a husband in the middle of his medical residency. It's hard. I've found that exercise, eating healthy, and sleep work wonders (go figure)."—Cami

Letting go of perfectionism and expectations is important to some patients.

"I have a motto. 'When it all gets too hard, simplify it.' I find most things can have a simpler version."—Lindy

"To keep myself from getting depressed about it, I just have to let some things go. I have to realize that I have hypothyroidism and I am not superwoman. I can't do it all and that's okay."—Melissa

"I've learned to let go of the idea of 'perfect' and evaluate my priorities."—Rose

A number of people reported that exercise was essential:

"I find that I actually have more energy throughout the day if I have exercised first thing in the morning. It's become absolutely necessary—if I don't, I'm toast."—Deborah

"What keeps me energized? The adrenaline from the daily duties that need to be done and my favorite . . . exercise!!! I love a hard cardio workout, and although I may be dead tired afterwards, it makes me feel wonderful!!"—Lisa

A number of patients have said that a good cry is a helpful first step when things are out of control.

"Sometimes, I need to cry for a minute. Breathe and let go of the stuff that can't get done. Then make a list in order of importance, start at the top, and do a little at a time with breaks when needed."—Kara

"I cry for a few minutes, do something just for me (paint nails, bath, short walk, etc.), let things go, say 'no' with love. Long term, daily exercise is a must. I insist (to myself) that I must start . . . after that, if I truly have nothing, I give myself permission to stop."—Holly

"I cry. Seriously, I do. It helps. I force myself to take walks and go to the park. I try to be social on those days as well. It helps me feel less alone and helps to banish my panic and blues. Those are also the days when the housework can go to hell. If I need a nap and my toddler will allow it,

I take a nap. I won't fight it, and I am a better person for it."—Stephanie

Having helpful family members is a tremendous help to many patients.

"The best thing you can have is support of your family. My husband is awesome. He does all the laundry and cooks and helps clean. When I feel yucky it helps to know I have a safe place that I won't be judged if I take a three-hour nap or stay in bed all morning."—Jen

"My kids have a chore chart and help me around the house. That helps when I'm feeling sluggish."—Jamie

"My husband steps in, makes dinner, and helps with laundry after working a long day. We have six children, so that meant a lot of pregnancies with me lying on the couch with undiagnosed Hashimoto's, feeling too tired and ill to live a normal life."—Rebecca

"I made sure that my family understands that kids, pets, and household are not ONLY a wife's duties!"—Cecilia

7

Doctor, Doctor, Give Me the News

Healing is a matter of time, but it is sometimes also a matter of opportunity.

—HIPPOCRATES

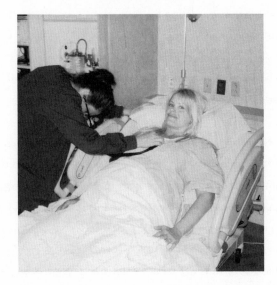

Before giving birth to Hudson Lee

Dealing with doctors and the whole medical system is such an important part of my own journey to wellness that I felt it deserved its own chapter.

As you can tell from my story, I spent a great deal of time going to different doctors, and I had my fair share of bad experiences.

I had doctors who told me my symptoms were in my head. I had doctors who told me there was nothing they could do, even though they had never run a thyroid test. I had doctors who were more interested in the fact that I'd been on television than in my health. I had doctors who leered at me. (Ick.) I can't tell you how many doctors never tested my thyroid or even put a hand on my neck! And I even had a doctor who refused to treat me, even after he knew I was hypothyroid.

I wasted so much time, and could have avoided so much suffering had I known then what I know now.

So, bear with me . . . I'm going to do some Monday-morning quarterbacking about dealing with doctors, and hopefully it will help you avoid making the mistakes I did.

KNOW YOUR FAMILY MEDICAL HISTORY

One of the most important things you can do is to know your family medical history.

I didn't know that we had a number of people in the family with thyroid disease. Had I known, I might have pushed far earlier for thyroid treatment.

Dr. Alan Christianson puts it in perspective: "In Gena's case, thyroid disease is pervasive in her family. For Gena, like many people with autoimmune thyroid disease, thyroid hormone output can be variable, you can see periods of hypothyroidism, followed by hyperthyroidism—and only after time does it become clear which direction the thyroid is going. In Gena's case, it became permanently underactive."

So make sure that you ask your parents, grandparents, and siblings about their health histories. If you have a family history of autoimmune disease or thyroid disease, make sure that you let each and every doctor know, and push for tests if you have suspicious symptoms.

DON'T ASSUME YOU HAVE TO BE
MIDDLE-AGED OR OLDER

I think one of the most important messages I want to get out is that you don't have to be forty, fifty, or older to get a thyroid condition. As you know from my own story, I suspect my thyroid problem started in my twenties.

Mary's thyroid condition started in her early thirties.

And we are definitely not alone.

Sherilyn is a twenty-one-year-old thyroid patient.

I was recently diagnosed with Hashimoto's six months ago, after quitting my job because I was struggling with depression. When I started my job, everything went to hell in a handbasket. I was severely depressed, I didn't sleep at night for fear of the morning coming and another shift starting at work. I cried every day after work in bed from the time I got home until I eventually fell asleep around 2 a.m. Everyone thought it was just me being afraid of my first job, and that it would eventually pass. Antianxiety pills and sleeping pills were what was "supposed" to keep me going until this "eventually passed." It didn't. I went to the doctor's office and he told me he would do a complete blood workup to see if it was depression or something else. Now I know I was one of the lucky ones. I was quickly found to have a thyroid antibody count of above 3,000, when the "normal" range was less than 20. My TSH was in the

400s. So it turned out I have Hashimoto's—an autoimmune disease—and hypothyroidism.

Elisha was a vibrant young woman in her twenties when she started experiencing debilitating fatigue.

It was the kind of fatigue that caused me to feel incredibly winded simply by walking up a few stairs, despite being an otherwise energetic person. Next, I started experiencing panic attacks, acne, dry skin, and migraines. At first, I blamed the symptoms on my stressful job and the fact that I was in the middle of planning my wedding. However, my instincts told me that they were all red flags, so I saw multiple doctors and complained to each of them about multiple hypothyroid and hyperthyroid symptoms that I had been experiencing. They consistently tested my TSH level and told me that it was "normal." Of course, I was naive and thought that doctors were all-knowing and heard several times, "You are just suffering from stress," and "Those are all normal signs of aging." (Even though I was in my twenties!) Frustrated and basically broke, I decided to take matters into my own hands. Combined with an educated guess and a leap of faith, I ordered my own blood tests and had them completed at my local LabCorp. The results were shocking; my anti-TPO antibodies were 272 and the entire panel of tests were outside of functional ranges for thyroid health. At the age of thirty, I finally obtained a diagnosis for what had been ailing me for years. I sought help from a doctor who practices integrative medicine, and he immediately started me on natural thyroid replacement. I adopted a gluten-free diet, and I'm finally on my way back to being my normal, healthy self.

Chris was in her early thirties and had symptoms for five years before she was finally diagnosed and treated for hypothyroidism.

When my daughter, now twenty-one, developed enlarged thyroid at the age of nine, I moved into action right away and had my pediatrician refer us to an endocrinologist, who started my daughter on levothyroxine. I am so committed to this that as a PhD nursing student, I am considering changing my focus to autoimmune thyroid disorder and interventions to improve symptom management!

Gina is only twenty-one, but after a severe thyroid storm—a life-threatening period of extreme hyperthyroidism—she feels like she's finally getting her life back.

Since I was in high school, I have been pretty sick. For the longest time no doctor could find anything wrong with me. My sophomore year was awful. I was constantly missing school, and it just got worse from there. About a year into college, I started getting the worst headaches and body pain every single day. I could never get up! I just wanted to sleep. Then I started to look sick. I was losing my hair and my weight just dropped out of nowhere! I went from an average weight of 130 pounds to close to 110. Because my weight dropped so dramatically people were getting concerned. Apparently, I had an attitude to match as well. I was always angry and crabby, and I couldn't control it. So I had to start defending that I didn't have an eating disorder. No one would believe me. After all this I had enough. I went to the doctor, who referred me to my first endocrinologist since my thyroid numbers were off. They had discovered that I had Graves' disease and severe hyperthyroidism.

Here I am now, at twenty-one years old and finally stable again. I am so grateful. It shows to never take life for granted and everyday is a miracle. I am so happy that I was given another chance. Please keep spreading the word about thyroid awareness for younger women. It can become so much more serious than people think!

DON'T BUY INTO THE THYROID STIGMA

My doctor, Alan Christianson, often says that thyroid disease is the "Rodney Dangerfield of medicine"—it gets no respect.

He's right. As he says, "A big part of the problem is the limitation of current thyroid testing and treatment. Patients end up being told—and believing—that whatever is wrong with them is their fault, so people are not open about it. They feel victimized."

So if you suspect you have a thyroid problem, or you've already been diagnosed, don't let doctors view you negatively.

If your doctor derisively tells you that your weight gain has nothing to do with your thyroid—as in, "get off the couch and get moving, and eat less!"—find another doctor.

If you have a doctor who whips out a prescription pad and wants to put you on an antidepressant no matter what thyroid symptoms you still have—get another doctor.

If your doctor who suggests that you only want a thyroid diagnosis as a way to lose weight—find another doctor.

I can't say it any more clearly. You deserve respect, and your thyroid treatment deserves respect. Any doctor not willing to give you that respect doesn't deserve your business, much less your trust.

ABOUT THOSE ENDOCRINOLOGISTS

Speaking of doctors, let's talk about endocrinologists.

While thyroid disease is within the expertise of the endocrinology specialty, let's be honest here. Endocrinologists can be essential for proper diagnosis and treatment of serious disease of the thyroid, such as thyroid cancer or life-threatening thyroid storm, as well as severe endocrine problems such as adrenal conditions like Cushing's disease and Addison's disease, osteoporosis, polycsytic ovary syndrome, and others. But they also typically treat diabetes—which, when improperly managed, can cause blindness, loss of limbs, and even death. Diabetes is on the rise in the United States. At the same time, we have a severe and worsening shortage of endocrinologists. Right now, there are an estimated 4,000 endocrinologists in the United States who are serving the 25 to 100 million Americans who might reasonably need to be seen by an endocrinologist. That's only one endocrinologist for every 6,250 to 25,000 people.

Given such a shortage, the endocrinologists are focusing their energy on diabetics and critical thyroid situations. And where does that leave women who don't feel well because of hypothyroidism or hormone imbalances? (I'm not suggesting that thyroid problems aren't serious.)

I'm definitely glad that I had a top-notch endocrinologist to evaluate my thyroid nodules and do the fine-needle aspiration biopsy. And I recommend that everyone with Hashimoto's or hypothyroidism have at least one consult with an endocrinologist, just to take a look at the gland's structure. But beyond that, my endocrinologist was not especially helpful.

Increasingly, even endocrinologists are leaving it to other physicians to diagnose and manage what they consider "routine" thyroid problems. And routine it is, at least to them. The American Association of Clinical Endocrinologists (AACE) says that keeping the thyroid in balance requires only "three easy steps"— TSH tests, taking a levothyroxine medication, and following up with a TSH test every six to twelve months. (By the way, been there, done that, and it didn't work for me!)

My advice? Unless you have what an endocrinologist would view as a "life-threatening" thyroid condition, look elsewhere for help.

But if you need to find a qualified endocrinologist, the AACE maintains an online Find an Endocrinologist database of clinical endocrinologists, by state. The American Thyroid Association (ATA) has a Find a Thyroid Specialist database featuring doctors who are members of the American Thyroid Association. The Endocrine Society's Hormone Foundation educational arm maintains a Find an Endocrinologist search function. Information on all these services is featured in the Resources section of this book.

FIND A KNOWLEDGEABLE DOCTOR

So how do you find that respectful, smart doctor to diagnose and treat hypothyroidism? They're not particularly easy to locate. Surprisingly in this day and age, there are still practitioners who actually believe that they can simply look at a patient and rule out thyroid disease. If you're not seriously overweight or middle-aged, if you've just had a baby, or your neck's not obviously enlarged, they may not even think you could be hypothyroid!

You probably will want to look beyond endocrinologists for your ongoing care and hypothyroidism treatment. As we've seen, endocrinologists tend to go totally by the book, which means annual TSH tests, levothyroxine, and a tendency to offer antidepressant prescriptions and ineffective advice for any other complaints you might have. Mary coached a woman who was a marathon runner and athlete and discovered that she was suddenly gaining weight. She also had every hypothyroid symptom in the book, a borderline hypothyroid TSH level, and elevated TPO antibodies. Did she get treatment from her endocrinologist? No. He told her she had "fork in mouth disease" and told her she needed to eat less and exercise more. Seriously, Doctor?

There are many different types of practitioners who have become effective at diagnosing, treating, and managing complex thyroid imbalances. They include some general practice or family practice doctors, internists, ob-gyns, nurse practitioners, antiaging medicine practitioners, bariatric physicians (specializing in weight loss), and osteopaths (DOs) as well as holistic and integrative practitioners—including holistic MDs, naturopaths (NDs), herbal medicine experts, and traditional Chinese medicine practitioners.

I probably saw more than twenty different doctors over the twenty years I was misdiagnosed, and it wasn't until I started seeing a naturopathic physician that I actually got the effective treatment I needed!

So how do you know which way to go?

First, think twice about using your general practitioner or family practice doctor. Many of them are forced to diagnose and treat thyroid disease, due to the endocrinologist shortage, but they are doing so without a great deal of knowledge or expertise. You can't assume that the thyroid treatment or hormone advice you are getting from a GP or family practice doctor is reflecting the best and most current thinking on the issue.

Many GPs and family doctors also rely on the laboratory report to flag abnormal results, which means that because most labs are still using the outdated TSH range, these doctors are usually not going to be aware that TSH levels above 2.5 to 3 may be indicative of thyroid problems.

Jacob Teitelbaum, MD, the expert on integrative medicine, says a more broad-minded practitioner is especially important for proper thyroid care: "General doctors don't do thyroid—they think they do thyroid, but they don't know how to do it properly. If you want it properly done, go to a holistic physician."

There are of course terrific doctors out there who follow a conventional approach. But if you're trying to find the right practitioner to partner with you for hormonal wellness, Mary and I both feel strongly that, if you can afford it, start by looking for a holistic/integrative practitioner who has a track record working with hormones.

By "holistic/integrative," we mean a practitioner—usually an MD, ND, or DO—who combines the best of conventional approaches with an open mind about other ways of diagnosing and treating conditions, and who has a working understanding of holistic, natural, and alternative medicine approaches. This is the sort of doctor who can help identify the best of all possible worlds for you in terms of your treatment.

The challenge is in how and where to find these practitioners, and, given that few of them are on insurance or available via HMOs, in paying for them.

To find these doctors, ask around. Ask friends, ask other holistic practitioners, ask at your local health food store, and if you
know a nurse, be sure to ask him or her. (Nurses are often very
clued in about the best doctors!)

Dr. Teitelbaum suggests starting with the American Board of
Integrative Holistic Medicine. ABIHM maintains a physician locator
service that can help you find more than 1,000 board-certified integrative and holistic doctors around the country. Contact information
for ABIHM is in the Resources section at the end of the book.

For lists of doctors who've been recommended by patients,
check the Thyroid Sexy website at http://www.thyroidsexy.com
and Mary Shomon's Thyroid Top Doctors Directory at http://
www.thyroid-info.com/topdrs.

As for affording these doctors, this can be a challenge. Because HMOs and health insurers only cover traditional treatment,
doctors who are covered by your insurance or who participate in
your HMO will probably be constrained by the rules of the organization, and only be able to offer you the basics—the TSH tests
and levothyroxine prescriptions. So, whenever possible, you may
have to save your pennies and do your best to afford at least one
consultation with a doctor who is known to be especially thyroid
savvy.

(But be smart about it. You can sometimes have your HMO or
insurance cover all the blood tests you may need.)

Claire is a thyroid patient who found that an integrative approach was essential:

My thyroid problem actually came about when I was very
young, twelve years old to be exact! I always had very poor
eating habits and had always been very tired and cranky. I

would come home from school and sleep until dinnertime, and then I would go right back to sleep after dinner and sleep all through the night until I had to get up in the morning. This nonsense went on for about a half a year, until my mom noticed and told me we needed to go figure out what was wrong. We suspected mono, and so did the doctor, but when the lab test came back my endocrinologist told me my thyroid was almost dead, and that I was the youngest case of Hashimoto's disease that he'd ever seen!

I struggled on Synthroid for the next seven years—with no information—until I got livid and started on a very long journey to heal. I went to any kind of doctor you can imagine, the best endocrinologists, family doctors, and nothing . . . I finally got somewhat of an answer when I went to a doctor that was a naturopath and MD and she told me natural thyroid would help. This was the first step that changed my life. This helped boost my quality of life. I then saw an expert who explained the dangers of gluten and food intolerances with Hashimoto's disease as well as the dangers of sugars that aren't found naturally. He put me on supplements to revive my digestive issues, my liver, and my insulin resistance. After six months, I felt like a million bucks. The final touch to get my disease under control is taking an adrenal supplement every single day so I don't suffer from adrenal fatigue.

The end result: eliminating gluten, dairy (not eggs), red meat, chicken, soy, exercising an hour a day six days a week, and feeling like I can take on whatever life throws at me next! I have come so far, and I'm now aspiring to be a naturopathic doctor myself, specializing in thyroid disorders, so I can spread this wonderful news to those who suffer as much as I did.

While naturopaths and other physicians who can prescribe medication offer options for thyroid patients, integrative physician David Borenstein, MD, says that thyroid patients should be careful about all the nondrug holistic "cures," "solutions," and "breakthroughs" being marketed for thyroid patients.

Marketing a program as a "drug-free" thyroid treatment is often a successful strategy that will attract patients who understandably wish to refrain from medicating, thinking there is another, more natural, alternative to manage their thyroid disorder. As an integrative medical physician, I completely understand this point of view, and in certain medical conditions, this is a sustainable option. In the case of complicated thyroid disorders, however, medication in the form of thyroid hormone is often an option that cannot be avoided, but rather required, in order to maintain proper health. For example, a patient who has had their thyroid surgically removed will not react to supplements. Patients who have had their thyroid chemically ablated by radioactive iodine for Graves' disease also fall into this category, and it takes carefully dosed medication and monitoring by a physician to stay on track. Lastly, pregnant women who are hypothyroid must ALWAYS opt for a physician to closely monitor their thyroid levels. The health of their pregnancy and unborn child depends on it.

DO YOUR RESEARCH BEFORE YOUR APPOINTMENT

Learn as much as you can before you even get to the doctor. The computer is my best friend—I can read other people's stories, get information, get the facts, formulate my questions, and be prepared before I go to a doctor's appointment.

Also remember that a doctor's appointment is really a business meeting. It's your job to keep on task. So as you're doing your research, make sure you write your questions down. You'll want to bring those questions with you to your appointment.

And don't be surprised if you discover that the doctor knows less than you do about a particular topic.

I remember the moment when I realized that medically, there is no Santa Claus! It was in the middle of a doctor's appointment, and I had mentioned something related to thyroid treatment. The doctor was backpedaling, and got huffy and puffy. I remember thinking, "Aha, I must be on to something."

It's disappointing, but it happens. If a doctor is inquisitive and really wants to be your partner, he'll usually ask questions or plan to do more research on his own when he comes up against something he doesn't know. If a doctor wants to shut you down, he'll get authoritarian or change the subject, or he'll even say something ridiculous, like "I'm the doctor, you're the patient."

That's your sign to head for the door!

At the same time, don't walk in with piles of papers to show the doctor. Dr. David Borenstein always encourages patients to do their homework before an appointment, and even to bring in relevant materials. "I have no problem with patients who come in with articles and research, unless it's going to take too much time from their visit. The most important part of the visit is for me to get to know the patient, listen to them and understand their symptoms. So, if it's done judiciously, that's fine. A couple of pages are fine. But reams of paper could take away from the patient's time and doesn't serve either of us."

BE SPECIFIC

One of the things that I've learned from Mary is how important it is as women to be as specific as possible with doctors, and to quantify your symptoms.

What do we mean by quantify? Well, what you do not want to do is to go in to the doctor and whine or complain. You know . . . "I'm just so tired, and I can't stand it." "Or, OMG, look at my rear end, it's huge. I feel like a blob." When they hear this sort of talk, doctors often turn off. They're hearing a whiny woman. And the advice tends to be pretty generic. "Sleep more, eat less, get more exercise" and so on.

But if you say, "Doctor, I am now sleeping ten hours a night instead of eight hours, and I'm still so exhausted that I need an hour's nap before I have the energy to make dinner," the doctor hears numbers, specifics, data upon which to make a diagnosis.

When you say, "I'm eating fifteen hundred calories per day on a low-fat diet, doing four hours a week of cardio, two hours of free weights, and I've been gaining at least two pounds a week for three months," again, that's information that a doctor hears not as whining, but as diagnostic data.

STAY CALM AND PROFESSIONAL

I have one piece of advice that is so important: Keep your cool, and be as unemotional as possible with the doctor.

If you become too emotional, the doctor starts to assume that your problems are stress and depression. If you lose your cool or get angry, that is just more evidence for the doctor that "She really is having emotional issues, not health problems."

There were times when I went in and just plain whined to doctors. And I always lost them. You can be persistent, but stay calm and keep it professional

BRING AN ADVOCATE WITH YOU

Many patients find it helpful to bring a spouse or trusted friend to appointments. Dr. David Borenstein says that this can often make for a more productive appointment. "I've found that it can be very helpful for patients to bring along someone they trust as an advocate. That person can help by asking questions that the patient might forget, and even take notes. I've even had an entire family sit in on an appointment."

STICK UP FOR YOURSELF WITH DOCTORS

Remember that when you see a doctor—whether it's with an HMO, or covered by your insurance, or you're paying out of pocket—YOU are the consumer, and they are the service provider. They are there to serve you. You are not there to sit meekly and accept everything the doctor has to say without question.

The typical doctor's visit lasts about seven minutes, and I've read that much of it is the doctor talking. Actually, they did these studies to see how long it takes the typical doctor before they interrupt the patient, and it was something like two or three seconds.

So you are going to have to stand your ground, and get the doctor to focus and listen.

My philosophy is, I'm paying for it, it's my time, and I'm going to make it worth every cent. I have my questions, and I don't leave until I get answers. If I get attitude instead of answers, or the doctor is looking at me like I have six heads, well, that's my last appointment here.

One thing about sticking up for yourself that I particularly wanted to mention is how often doctors refuse to even run thyroid tests. If it was your idea to have it tested, they may push back out of insecurity or ego. Some thoroughly confused doctors think that anyone who asks for a thyroid test is looking for weight loss pills.

And there are some doctors who are just plain clueless when it comes to thyroid issues. Believe it or not, at our Thyroid Sexy community, we've heard from patients whose doctors refused to run thyroid tests. The reasons?

> "You're only in your twenties [or thirties]. Only old people get
>   thyroid disease."
> "You just had a baby, and people with thyroid problems can't
>   get pregnant."
> "You just had a baby. It's postpartum depression."
> "You're just looking for an excuse for being overweight."
> "You're fat, and you think that thyroid pills will help you lose
>   weight."
> "You're just stressed out. Try to relax."
> "You just have PMS."
> "It's just age. Of course you're exhausted. What do you expect
>   at fifty [or sixty or seventy]?"

Are you appalled yet? I am, every time I hear one of these stories.

Of course, there's also my personal favorite: "You're depressed. Here's an antidepressant prescription." I seem to have run into my fair share of these doctors! And yet, did you know that some researchers estimate that at least 15 percent of those di-agnosed with depression are actually suffering from undiagnosed hypothyroidism? And on the antidepressant prescribing informa-tion—you know, the tiny print insert they give you with your prescription—it says that thyroid tests should be run BEFORE the physician prescribes antidepressants. Hah!

One thing that you can do is to bring a Thyroid Risks and Symptoms Checklist with you to your appointment. You can find one at www.thyroid-info.com. Bring an extra copy, and that way, you and the doctor can have the evidence right in front of you.

If your doctor reviews your checklist and refuses to order thyroid tests, you can write a letter that states the various reasons you have requested thyroid testing and the fact that this doctor has refused. Send the letter to the HMO or the insurance ombudsman. Sometimes this will get things moving.

Mary has a tip that, so far, has always worked. She recom-mends that you ask that a copy of your risks and symptoms check-list be added to your medical chart, after the doctor signs and dates it and notes that he or she has read it and discussed it with you. Ask for a signed copy for yourself.

As you can imagine, most doctors will not document that they refused you a test, because it could come back to haunt them if you were in fact diagnosed later. So you'll probably get the tests you need.

And if the doctor actually signs it, but still refuses to do the tests, send a copy to the HMO or insurance company's consumer liaison, along with your request that testing be performed.

Yes, it's playing hardball, but sometimes you have to do this to work around all the ridiculous hurdles doctors, HMOs, and in-surers put in front of us.

IF DOCTORS WON'T DO IT,
ORDER YOUR OWN TESTS

If you are unable to get your own physician to order the tests you need, remember that you do have another option. In most states, you can legally have any blood tests you need done through a patient-directed testing service. These services allow you to pick the blood tests you want, pay for them out of pocket—usually at costs that are close to the wholesale rate and not the marked-up rates that doctors charge. You can then go to a local branch of a nationally certified lab to have your blood drawn. The difference is, the results are sent back to *you*.

At that point, you can use this information in your search for a new doctor, or you may be able to show these results to your current doctor and get him or her to take further action. The lab that Mary has used for years is MyMedLab. More information is available in the Resources section.

Part 3

GOING FORWARD

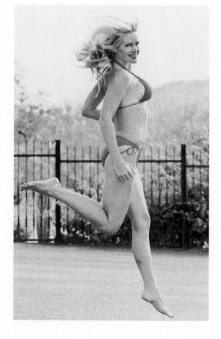

8

Weight Challenges:
How to Be the Biggest Loser

Never go to excess, but let moderation be your guide.
—CICERO

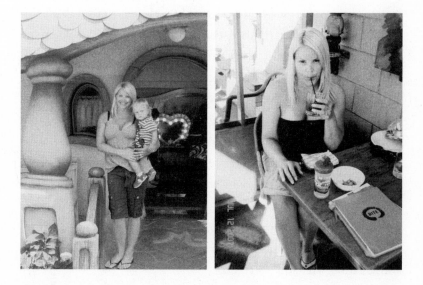

It's such a common complaint, and one that has frustrated me along the way—remember my delightful two days at *Celebrity Fit Club*? Well, we decided that it's worth dedicating a whole chapter to the issue of weight loss for thyroid patients, because it's what so many of us are talking about and struggling to resolve.

As you know, ups and downs in weight have been a struggle

for me, and I now know that a lot of that was due to my undiagnosed thyroid problem. There is so much misinformation out there about the link between thyroid and weight gain, but let me tell you one important thing: having an underactive thyroid can make you gain weight—even a great deal of weight—and it can make it hard, or even impossible, to lose weight. Any doctor who tells you that it isn't so is not paying attention.

Some doctors will tell you that hypothyroidism can't cause more than a few pounds of weight gain. That's a myth. One of the major complaints from our community members is that they started out at a perfectly normal weight and then started to pile on weight quickly—at rates that seem almost impossible!—when the thyroid problem began. Even after treatment, they have a tough time losing it.

And remember, even after you get on the right thyroid treatment, that doesn't mean the weight melts off. It's more likely that after starting thyroid medication, you'll lose a few pounds, usually water weight, as the water retention of hypothyroidism starts to abate, then it's up to you—what you eat, and how much you move—to keep the scale moving in the right direction. When it comes to maintaining or losing weight as a thyroid patient, unfortunately, there is no celebrity secret—I wish there were, but it's all about eating well and exercising.

We've put together a sort of crash course on the most important things to know about the thyroid and your weight challenges. It's all the things I wish I knew twenty years ago, when my thyroid first went haywire!

THYROID, HORMONES, AND MEDICAL ISSUES

Optimize Your Thyroid Treatment

I can't emphasize enough how important it is to make sure your hypothyroidism is diagnosed and your treatment is optimized. As I outlined before, that usually means that your TSH level is under 2, and your free T4 and free T3 levels are in the upper half of the reference range. Ultimately, many of us need to add some form of T3, or switch to a natural thyroid drug, to get things into optimal range. Also make sure your reverse T3 isn't elevated, and if it is, work with a practitioner—usually with adrenal support and supplemental T3—to get these levels down.

Believe me, if you don't optimize your treatment, you can work out hours a day and eat almost nothing, but you'll most likely be wasting your time, and you might even end up gaining more weight! (Mary and I both speak from experience.)

Getting optimized doesn't make the weight just fall off magically, of course. (Too bad . . . because it would be nice if it did!) But it does make it far more likely that following a healthy diet and exercise will finally start to work when it didn't before.

Test for and Treat Leptin Resistance

I don't want to forget to mention the leptin test. This is a blood test that I never knew about before becoming a thyroid patient. As it turns out, leptin is a hormone that sends messages between the brain and metabolism about your food intake, delivering instructions about the need to store—or burn—fat. When it all works, after you eat, the right amount of leptin is released, and then your body gets the message, "Hey, you, you have enough fat stored now to avoid starvation, so stop eating!" That "stop eating" message is translated into a reduction in appetite, metabolism speeds up, fat is burned, and leptin levels drop back to normal.

But sometimes this mechanism gets fouled up, and the cells don't listen. You eat, the leptin is released, but the message isn't received and more leptin is released. It's shouting, "Stop eating!" But the message isn't getting through. You're still hungry, your cells keep storing fat, and you never shift into fat-burning mode. It's a recipe for weight loss disaster!

Thyroid and hormone experts Kent Holtorf, MD, and Sara Gottfried, MD, regularly test leptin levels in any thyroid patient who is gaining weight or who can't lose weight. They both feel that the levels should ideally be under 10.

If the levels are elevated, you may want to take some steps specifically to improve leptin sensitivity and lower leptin levels, including stress reduction, getting enough sleep, moderate exercise, avoiding large meals, eliminating sugar and processed carbohydrates, eating three regular meals a day without snacking in between, and not eating after 8 p.m., to allow the body to reset toward more fat burning.

Dr. Holtorf has also found that injectible type 2 diabetes drugs like Symlin, Byetta, and Victoza—along with a carbohydrate-controlled diet—may help counteract leptin resistance.

Test for and Treat Insulin Resistance

Consider getting your glucose—blood sugar—tested. At a minimum, you can get a glucose level from a home test kit, but preferably, get a fasting glucose to evaluate whether your blood sugar is normal, high normal, or elevated. In late 2003, the American Diabetes Association recommended that the cutoff level for "pre-diabetes" be changed to 100 mg/dl, down from 110 mg/dl. This meant that levels above 100 mg/dl are considered evidence of insulin resistance, on the way to type 2 diabetes. And insulin resistance makes it harder to lose weight.

If your levels come back above 100, you may want to take some actions to help prevent progression to type 2 diabetes, including:

- Reducing or eliminating simple carbohydrates, refined grains, processed foods, diet sodas, artificial sweeteners
- Regularly exercising
- Getting sufficient sleep—at least seven to eight hours a night
- Managing daily stress
- Stopping smoking

Ron Rosedale, MD, has a website with a very straightforward eating plan that can help reverse insulin resistance. It basically eliminates grains, fruit, and sugar, focuses on lean proteins, vegetables, nuts, and good fats. It's similar to—and a bit more demanding—than some of the new "paleo" diets, but it seems to work well for many people.

Some practitioners are also having success using several type 2 diabetes medications to prevent progression of insulin resistance to full diabetes. The medications include the pill metformin (Glucophage) and injectible medications including pramlintide (Symlin), exenatide (Byetta), and Victoza (Liraglutide).

If you do take metformin, you should know that there are some studies that showed that metformin can suppress TSH levels. Patients who were hypothyroid and taking metformin had very low TSH levels—it looked like they should be hyperthyroid, but they had no signs or symptoms of hyperthyroidism, and their free T4 and free T3 levels were normal. So TSH tests alone aren't reliable for thyroid patients on metformin.

Test and Optimize Vitamin D Levels

Vitamin D is not just a vitamin we now know it's a hormone and that it's important for immune function and weight loss. So you'll want to get it tested—your doctor can run the blood test or you can order it yourself if needed. Many of the doctors we talk to like to see thyroid patients with vitamin D levels above 50 (on the typical range of around 20 to 100) for optimal health. Talk to your doctor about where she/he would like you to be in vitamin D levels. (And a tip—best time to take your vitamin D is with dinner—not in the morning!)

Test for and Treat Candidiasis/Yeast Overgrowth

Thyroid patients are more susceptible to developing candidiasis— that's a chronic overgrowth of the fungus *Candida*—also known as yeast. A yeast overgrowth can make it harder to lose weight.

If you did a long-term course of antibiotics, eat a lot of sugar, or have used steroids, you're at much higher risk for developing yeast overgrowth. Symptoms are:

- Frequent vaginal yeast, genital yeast, including "jock itch," and athlete's foot infections
- Frequent oral yeast infections (thrush)
- Frequent infections of the nipple/breast when breast-feeding
- Chronic ear, upper respiratory, allergic, or sinus problems

- Urticaria (hives, wheals, or welts); itching or burning skin
- Stomach, digestive, and elimination problems
- Fluid retention, swelling, and bloating
- Difficulty losing weight, or inappropriate weight gain

These are just a few of the dozens of other symptoms attributed to *Candida* overgrowth. Your doctor can run a blood test, called a *Candida* immune complex assay test, a stool test, or a *Candida* culture, to confirm its presence. Treating a yeast overgrowth is more complicated, however. Typically, doctors recommend dietary changes to eliminate foods that contain or feed yeast—bread, sugars, fruit, dairy, mushrooms, fermented foods—adding probiotics, antiyeast supplements, and, for stubborn cases, prescription antifungal drugs like fluconazole (Diflucan), terbinafine hydrochloride (Lamisil), nystatin (Nystan), and itraconazole (Sporanox).

Consider Supplements

You may want to try supplements to help with weight loss. Be careful with stimulants and with supplements that contain caffeine or guarana—they may be counterproductive and tire out the adrenals.

We suggest that for combination weight loss supplements, you stick with the experts. Kent Holtorf, MD, an expert on hormone balance and weight loss, has formulated some specialized supplements to help with blood sugar and metabolism, as part of his Holtraceuticals line. Ann Louise Gittleman, ND, also has some excellent weight loss formulas as part of her Fat Flush program.

Lately, Mary swears by raspberry ketones and Sweet Wheat, a form of wheatgrass, which both seem to help her.

Some other supplements that may help with weight loss in

various ways—suppressing appetite, balancing blood sugar, increasing metabolism, blocking fat—include:

Acetyl-L-carnitine

Alpha-lipoic acid

Calcium

Caralluma fimbriata

Chromium

Coenzyme Q-10

DHEA

Fat blockers and starch blockers—i.e., chitosan, *Phaseolus vulgaris*

Glucosol

Glutamine/L-glutamine

Hoodia gordonii

Irvingia (sometimes known as wild mango, African mango)

Milk thistle

Pantethine

Pyruvate

Spirulina

Taurine

Mary's *Thyroid Diet Revolution* goes through each of these supplements in detail and explains what they do and why you may want to consider taking them. There is also information at www .thyroid-info.com.

Consider Weight Loss Drugs

Some physicians are finding that combining the antiaddiction and immune-modulating drug naltrexone, along with the antidepressant bupropion, is helpful for weight loss. Right now, combining these medications is considered an off-label treatment—meaning that it's not an FDA-approved use of these drugs—but it's legal for physicians to prescribe them in this manner. Down the road, drug manufacturers are hoping to get FDA approval for a drug, Contrave, that combines the two in one pill.

Kent Holtorf, MD, regularly uses these two drugs together to help his patients with weight loss.

> I've found that the antidepressant Wellbutrin (bupropion) does not work well for weight loss. A combination of Wellbutrin and low-dose naltrexone (LDN) is, however, having some surprisingly good results. Typically, we have the patients on 300 mg of Wellbutrin-SR twice a day, along with an increasing dose of naltrexone, typically 10, up to 20, and then to 30. At a lower dose, for example 4½ mg daily, it helps as an immune modulator, and at higher doses it seems to help with weight, cravings, and the set point.

You've probably also heard about the drug Alli, which is available over-the-counter, and in higher doses by prescription as Xenical; the generic name is orlistat. This drug helps remove some of the dietary fat from food. You should know that it also can interfere to some extent with your ability to absorb your medication. And to be honest, we haven't heard from any thyroid patients who have successfully lost weight using this drug. But we have heard from patients who have had all sorts of really unpleasant side effects when trying it, including what patients call "Alli Oops," the uncontrollable diarrhea and accidental leakage—sometimes in public—that can result from eating too much fat while taking the drug. No, thanks . . .

Cryotherapy

I also wanted to mention cryotherapy, a very interesting treatment that Dr. Alan Christianson is using to help with metabolism and weight gain. He regularly tests women who are struggling with weight and finds that they're only burning 800 to 900 calories a day. No one can lose weight if that's all their body needs to function in a day—you can't eat less than that and still get proper nutrition. It's not even safe. That's where cryotherapy comes in.

I'll let Dr. Christianson explain:

With hypothyroidism, there is often suppression of metabolism, weight gain, fatigue, pain, and poor response to exercise. Cryotherapy was pioneered in the early 1970s by Japanese scientists, and has been big in Europe for decades, but only recently has it started to be used in the U.S., mainly for athletes. Cryotherapy burns calories and reduces inflammation. The abrupt drop of temperature—in whole body cryotherapy, the skin is exposed to a very brief blast of temperatures of −250°F—has huge metabolic repercussions. The neurologic response is that the body is hardwired to deal with freezing. In cryotherapy, the patient stands in a chamber, with the head outside the chamber. Liquid nitrogen chills to the target temperature, circulates around the body, and causes the nervous system to raise metabolism and excrete inflammatory chemicals. Even after a three-minute treatment, we can see reduction in swollen joints, and via calorimetry, we can see an increase in metabolism.

A single session of cryotherapy spurs a dramatic reaction. In the hours following the treatment, they typically burn 500 to 800 extra calories, with a lasting increase of 200 to 250 calories a day for as long as three weeks. After multiple treatments, I've seen patients reset their basal metabolic rate to more normal levels, along with seeing an increase in energy.

I've tried it, and even though it sounds strange, it's not at all uncomfortable, and you don't walk out feeling particularly cold. And it does seem to help pump up my metabolism. Hey, you try everything, right?!

Evaluate Your Medications

While you should never stop taking any medications without your doctor's direction, you'll want to know if your medications may be making weight loss more difficult. Here is a partial list of some medications that can cause or promote weight gain:

Steroids (i.e., prednisone)
Estrogen and progesterone independently, together as the Pill,
    or together in hormone therapy
Antidiabetic drugs, like insulin
Various antidepressants, especially Prozac, Paxil, and Zoloft

Mood stabilizers and anticonvulsants like lithium, valproate
   (Depakote), and carbamazepine (Tegretol)
Beta-blockers
Sedatives and tranquilizers

In some cases, there are options that may cause less weight gain, so it's worth a discussion with your doctor.

Especially for People with Hypothyroidism

No matter which plan you choose, when you are following a weight loss program, there are some things we people with hypothyroidism need to remember.

It's not going to happen quickly. Sure, we all want to drop five pounds in a week, but that's just not how it works for most thyroid patients. If you lose a pound in a week, that's GREAT. Don't compare your diet success to other people's—and especially not your metabolically gifted friends'—or you'll make yourself depressed and frustrated. Just compete with yourself! (Mary always tells people to remember that a pound of fat is four sticks of butter—so think about that the next time you see you're down a pound on the scale!)

Another thing is, you are going to have to exercise. Some people can lose weight and maintain it without working out, but for thyroid patients, it's really not an option. You're going to need to build muscle—because it helps raise your metabolism—and do some aerobic activity, because it helps burn calories.

Keep in mind that fiber is really important and helpful for thyroid dieters, but if you add a significant amount of fiber to your diet, you should have your thyroid levels rechecked in about eight weeks, because fiber can change your absorption, and you may need a different dosage.

Finally, if you lose more than 10 percent of your body weight, YOU ROCK! (My advice? Go buy a new pair of smaller jeans to celebrate!) But, don't forget that it's also time to get retested to see if you need to adjust your dosage of thyroid medication.

WHAT YOU EAT AND DRINK— MAJOR CHANGES

Yes, you've heard all about my love of the Melting Pot and Big Macs, but most of the time, I do try to eat well. If I am not careful about what I eat, the weight can easily start to pile on.

There are two major changes that Mary and I are both making and that we've found helpful. First, we have both made the decision to go gluten free and avoid wheat and gluten products. Not only does that help inflammation, but it also helps one keep weight down in general. We've replaced the traditional bread, cereals, crackers, and snacks with gluten-free versions and alternatives.

I've also followed the example of my friend Alec Baldwin and eliminated sugar. Alec recently dropped thirty pounds simply by avoiding sugar, and he looks and feels great.

The Gluten-Free Diet

Eating gluten free means eliminating gluten, a protein that is found in grains such as wheat, rye, and barley. Yes, that means no traditional bread, pasta, cereal, and such. (But the good news is that gluten-free versions of all the foods we love are popping up more and more often.)

Eating gluten free is essential treatment for people who have the autoimmune condition known as celiac disease—also called celiac sprue or celiac sprue-dermatitis.

Celiac disease is a serious chronic disease that causes the digestive system to be unable to absorb nutrients from food. If you have celiac disease, your intestinal lining becomes inflamed, and eventually destroyed, by exposure to gluten. This makes you unable to digest and absorb nutrients, and can cause a variety of immune dysfunctions or trigger certain autoimmune diseases, including autoimmune Hashimoto's or Graves' disease. And celiac disease is as much as thirty times more common in autoimmune patients.

The main noninvasive way to diagnose celiac disease is a blood test that measures antibodies to gluten—antigliadin, antiendomysium, and antireticulin. There's also a home or office finger-prick test that does an analysis known as an IgA tissue transglutaminase (tTG). In some cases, doctors need to run an endoscope into your bowels to take a look—or do a biopsy—and make an accurate diagnosis.

Some people do not have full celiac disease, yet they are sensitive to gluten. This also seems to be far more common in autoimmune patients, and the condition is on the rise. While full celiac disease often causes weight loss, gluten intolerance seems more likely to cause weight gain, due to chronic inflammation.

Symptoms of celiac disease and gluten intolerance/sensitivity include:

Diarrheal, watery, odorous stools
Abdominal bloating, cramps, excessive or explosive gas
Weight loss or gain
Weakness, fatigue, including muscle weakness
Bone pain

Tingling and numbness in hands and feet

Absence of menstrual periods, delayed start of menstrual
periods in adolescents

Infertility in women and men

Orthostatic hypotension, where your blood pressure drops and
you feel dizzy or faint when you stand up or get out of bed

If you have celiac disease, it's crucial that you stay on a strict gluten-free diet for life, to prevent damage and complications from the disease. Your doctor, books, and support groups can help.

If you are gluten intolerant, avoiding or eliminating gluten can be an important part of staying healthy, and can help you in the weight loss battle. We've heard from many thyroid patients who have found that even though they were not diagnosed with celiac disease, they lost weight, felt less fatigued, got rid of bloating, and reduced their thyroid medication dosage after adopting a gluten-free diet.

Some of Our Favorite Gluten-Free Products

(See the Resources section for websites and contact information.)

- Chex Gluten Free Cereals—low in sugar, great for kids
- Udi's Bakery—all sorts of products, bagels, breads, etc.
- Nut Thins crackers—these are light, rice crackers in all sorts of flavors, like barbecue, ranch, sea salt—wonderful!
- Pamela's gluten-free products—great pancakes and baking products
- Mary's Gone Crackers crackers—delicious, nutty flavor and great crunch

The Low-Glycemic Diet

I mentioned that Alec Baldwin cut out sugar. There's actually a term for this type of eating—it's called "low-glycemic." And it's actually a really good way to fight insulin resistance, calm inflammation, and lose weight for some thyroid patients in particular.

High-glycemic foods are the sugary, starchy foods—anything made with white flour—plus anything made with sugar. What's left to eat? Actually, quite a few things: low-fat protein sources (like chicken, turkey, fish, lean red meats, nuts, lower-fat dairy); nonstarchy, high-fiber vegetables and fruits; and good fats.*

If you avoid sugar in all forms and emphasize lean sources of protein, some good fat, nonstarchy vegetables, with limited fruit and eat starches, which when consumed on ocassion are high in fiber, you are on your way toward a low-glycemic diet.

It's a commitment to follow a low-glycemic diet—and you have to rethink some of your typical ways of eating—but it may just be the change you need.

WHAT YOU EAT AND DRINK— THINGS TO CONSIDER

There are so many things to keep in mind when it comes to what you eat and drink to lose weight. Some steps to take:

---

*Remember that these high-fiber vegetables are also goitrogenic, meaning that they promote thyroid enlargement and can potentially cause or aggravate hypothyroidism. Cooking or steaming eliminates most of their goitrogenic properties.

Avoid Toxins: Eat organic, pesticide-free, and hormone-free foods whenever possible.

Avoid Allergens: Eliminate foods you're allergic or sensitive to. For me, that's wheat/gluten. Others may need to eliminate dairy or soy, for example.

Don't Go Soy Crazy: Lots of diet programs rely on soy-heavy meal substitutes, and many diet shakes, snacks, and bars have a high amount of soy, which may block thyroid absorption, and even slow down the thyroid in some cases. So you probably want to stay away from soy-based diet plans and products. And for soy in general: don't overdo it, especially with processed soy products, soy milk, or soy supplements.

Get Enough Fiber: Aim to get 25 to 30 grams of fiber per day, ideally from foods. Fiber is essential to digestion and optimizing your weight loss efforts. Fiber has minimal calories but can fill you up by adding bulk, and when consumed with carbohydrates, it helps modulate the insulin response and normalize blood sugar. Remember that if you switch from a low-fiber to a high-fiber diet, you'll want to have your thyroid levels rechecked within two months to see if you need a dosage readjustment. Some of the highest-fiber foods are beans, broccoli, cabbage, greens (like collards, kale, turnip greens), spinach, and sweet potatoes.

Eat Enough Protein, and Shift to Lower-Fat Protein Sources: Protein is needed to build muscle (which raises metabolism) and to maintain your energy level, and so your food intake should include sufficient levels of protein. Ideally, include a portion of lean protein as part of every meal and snack, and never eat a carbohydrate—whether vegetable, fruit, or starch—without an accompanying protein, because it helps slow down the digestion of the carbohydrate as it converts to sugar. If you are a beef eater, try switching to the lower-fat cuts, like filet, top round, and London broil. Better yet, consider buffalo, a high-protein, low-fat red meat. If you're eating poultry, focus on white versus dark meat. When you do eat beef or poultry, try to use organic, hormone-free, grass-fed meat and free-range poultry whenever possible, and trim visible fat. Consider substituting more seafood, beans, and nuts for meat and poultry.

Shop the Outside of Your Food Store: The way food stores are laid out, the vegetables, meats, and healthier foods are in the outer areas, while the processed and sugary packaged foods are in the center aisles. That's why many nutrition experts say we should shop the perimeter! There are also great stores like Trader Joe's and Whole Foods, where you are much more likely to find all sorts of healthy options and choices in every aisle.

Incorporate Good Fats: You want to minimize or eliminate the saturated and trans fats found in fatty cuts of red meat, full-fat dairy products, many fried foods, and many processed foods. Instead, focus on polyunsaturated and monounsaturated fats—for example, those found in nuts, oily fish, avocados, olive oil, and canola oil.

Drink Lots of Water: Only when the body has taken in sufficient water can body temperature be maintained for optimal metabolism. Dehydration can make the body temperature drop slightly, and with a reduction in temperature, the body will attempt to help raise temperature by storing fat to act as an insulator. So, drinking too little water can contribute to an inefficient metabolism and hoarding of fat. Also, hypothyroidism can both cause water retention and bloating. It may sound counterintuitive, but if you're bloated or retaining water, one of the best things you can do is drink more water. Water also aids in digestion and elimination. Mary and I both like Smart Water and the other electrolyte-enhanced waters. Somehow, they seem to be absorbed really well. But any good-quality filtered water will do. (Some experts recommend that you drink as much as one ounce of water for every pound of your current body weight. Most of us would end up floating away, but hey, it's worth a try!)

Watch the Goitrogens: Don't go overboard on raw goitrogenic veggies. These are the vegetables that are great for you, but when raw—or juiced—can slow down your thyroid. So watch those spinach and kale smoothies, and don't go on the "all-cabbage" diet. But if you steam or lightly cook these vegetables, and don't eat them for breakfast, lunch, and dinner daily, it shouldn't be a problem.

Be Careful with Coffee and Tea: Coffee is controversial. Some studies show that it helps reduce blood sugar and insulin sensitivity and reduces the risk of type 2 diabetes. Coffee also has caffeine, which is proven to raise metabolism. But at the same time, there are studies that show that coffee can raise blood sugar in the short term, trigger a stress response, and cause abdominal weight gain. If you're trying to lose weight, it probably makes sense to stick to a cup or two a day—and no, a "venti" or grande or extra-large is not a cup! Keep track of how you feel after you've had coffee, because if you notice that you feel shaky, or hungry, then that's a sign to cut back. Tea drinkers—including our iced tea friends—also be careful because black tea is high in fluoride and may be a problem. Want to drink something that might help? Consider green tea. Apparently, people who drink five cups of green tea a day typically burn 80 more calories over a twenty-four-hour period. Green tea has a fat-burning ingredient, epigallocatechin gallate—or EGCG—that's also found in a lot of diet supplements.

Eliminate Most Sweeteners—Artificial or Otherwise: At our thyroid community, some people say, "I've switched from sugar to agave," or "I use honey and not sugar anymore," but in the end, these sorts of changes aren't necessarily going to help in the diet area. Ideally, you should avoid all sweeteners entirely, whether white and brown table sugars, molasses, honey, maple syrup, agave, or corn syrup. This also goes for the so-called "healthier" sweeteners, like sorbitol, mannitol, xylitol, and maltitol. As for artificial, low- or no-calorie sweeteners (you know, the pink packets, blue packets, and yellow packets) including those in diet sodas, we now know that they may actually sabotage our efforts to lose weight. It turns out that artificial sweeteners train the body that sweetness is "false" and doesn't require a fat-burning response. So this can mean that when you do eat something that has sweetness WITH calories, the automatic response doesn't kick in, metabolism doesn't go up, and fat is not burned. Low- and no-calorie artificial sweeteners train your body to overconsume (and store) carbohydrates! (Uh-oh! I'd better go dump that diet soda right this minute!) If you need a sweetener, most of the holistic nutritional folks suggest that you try stevia. It has no calories, and unlike other sweeteners, seems to improve insulin sensitivity slightly.

Watch Fruit and Fructose: Fruit is controversial, especially for thyroid patients, because some of us simply cannot lose weight when we have fruit in our diet. Fruit is high in fructose, a type of sugar that is easily and quickly converted into body fat. (We all know about the high-fructose corn syrup—half glucose and half fructose—found in processed and fast foods.) It turns out that the liver is not effective preventing fructose from being converted to fat—as compared to glucose. So, step one: if you see high fructose corn syrup listed as a packaged food or drink's ingredient, just drop that item from your food list. Apple juice, pear juice, and apple cider are juices from higher-fructose fruits, so you may want to limit them or avoid them entirely. Also watch your intake of pears, cherries, peaches, plums, grapes, dates, prunes, and apples, as these fruits are highest in fructose.

Limit Alcohol: Alcohol is empty calories, and whether it's a part of your diet plan is going to be up to you. If you do choose to drink, the heart-healthiest option is a glass of red wine. Make it a point to avoid liqueurs and cordials and frozen restaurant drinks—like margaritas—which can have hundreds of calories a glass and are usually loaded with sugar. Alcohol may slow, or even stall, your weight loss effort, so if you think you are doing everything right, but you're still not losing weight, try even a week or two without any alcohol and see if it gets the scale moving again.

HOW AND WHEN YOU EAT

Many of us rush around so much, we end up wolfing down our food. Then the brain doesn't get the message that we've eaten, we're full, and we can shift from storing fat to burning fat. So make sure that you chew your food well. The process of chewing starts the hormonal process of digesting the food, and helps the message reach the brain that you are eating, and getting full.

It's also a good idea to avoid large meals in general and avoid overeating at a meal. Good advice, and not always easy to follow, especially if you're eating out. One tip: avoid restaurants that offer "endless" pasta bowls and steer clear of buffets and "all-you-can-eat" places. (I do make an exception for pregnant women who want to visit the Melting Pot, however!)

Timing is also important. Try to finish your dinner at least three to four hours before you go to bed, and avoid eating after dinner (or after 8 p.m.), including bedtime snacks. This lets your body shift into fat-burning mode. Then, do your best to allow ten to twelve hours between dinner and breakfast. This makes the overnight period even more productive at fat burning. If you can, don't snack between meals and allow five to six hours between meals. Again, this allows the body to shift from storing fat into burning fat. If you are constantly eating—grazing, mini-meals, and so on—your body thinks that food is always around the next corner (because it is!) and never feels the need to shift into fat burning.

Mindful Eating

One of the most important things you can start doing today is mindful eating. What we mean is getting away from that sort of eating where you barely chew before you swallow, you're multitasking, or you're so distracted—by driving, the television, phone, computer, or something you're reading—that you can barely remember eating.

When you eat mindfully, you eat thoughtfully and slowly. You look at the food. You smell it. You taste it. And it actually helps your body and hormones respond appropriately to the food, to have pleasure from what you eat, and to activate the fat-burning hormones that metabolize it.

There are all sorts of studies that show that eating quickly, as compared to slowly, curtails the release of hormones that induce feelings of being full. The faster you eat, the less satisfied you'll feel.

So eat slowly and mindfully. Don't eat while standing, reading, driving, watching television, or texting. If you're not paying attention, your brain and body may not get the message that you've actually eaten.

LIFESTYLE ISSUES

Keep Track of What You Eat

It may sound silly, but actually writing down what you're eating can be a help. The act of writing it down makes you more aware and likelier to make better choices. Get a little notebook for your purse, or use an app on your smartphone . . . it doesn't matter what form it takes, it's the action of sitting down and thinking about your goals, what you're going to eat, and assessing what you've eaten that makes the difference.

Get More Sleep

Did you know studies show that it's almost impossible to lose weight if you get less than seven to eight hours of sleep a night? One doctor even told me that you're better off sleeping in the morning if you want to lose weight than getting up early for an exercise session! Hmmm . . . now, that's my kind of doctor!

Practice Active Stress Reduction

Active stress reduction means something that really relaxes the whole nervous system, like nonstrenuous yoga, breathing, or meditation. (It does not mean a pint of Ben & Jerry's on the couch while watching television!)

When you don't manage stress, you flood your body with cortisol—the stress hormone that also stimulates appetite. At the same time, the increased adrenaline increases fatty acid and blood sugar levels, which triggers the body to store extra calories primarily as fat in your abdominal area—the worst place to gain weight from a health standpoint. The abdominal fat makes you more insulin resistant and produces various inflammatory markers that increase your risk of diabetes, insulin resistance, and heart disease. It's a vicious circle.

So, one of the most important parts of successful weight loss is to incorporate active stress reduction into your daily life. By active stress reduction, we're not talking about "relaxing" as many of us think of it. Reading or watching television can be relaxing. But here, we are talking about specific activities that can help lower heart and respiration rates, reduce stress hormones, and help your energy, immune system, and overall health.

What you do depends on you. Some people like to do meditation, prayer, guided imagery, breathing exercises, or biofeedback. Others find yoga, tai chi, or a solitary walk on the beach helpful. Some people find that working with their hands—sewing, knitting, crocheting, gardening, kneading bread—gives them that sort of stress reduction. Whatever you do, make sure that you do some each day.

STAYING FIT, OR GETTING FIT

All right, I'm not one to jump for joy about going to the gym, but I have to say I've always felt my best when I exercise. I try to maintain a three-day-a-week regimen that consists of thirty minutes on the treadmill, light weights, and core work. If weather permits, I'll go for a run. If that's too much, I'll start off with a brisk walk to get the blood flowing. Remember, this is all predicated on how I'm feeling at the time. I listen to my body, and that always leads the way.

The key is finding something you like to do, because if it's not fun, you just won't stick with it. (I won't even bother to tell you about my one and only Spinning class, for example.)

I also try to fit in as much activity as I can—when I have the energy—by doing things like going for a walk or ride with the children or playing at the park.

And there have been times when exercise was entirely out of the question. I was too tired, achy, and burned out to do more than what I needed simply to get through the day.

But I'll tell you, there's nothing better than the feeling after a good workout! And I like to eat. As you know, I've had to lose extra baby weight multiple times after pregnancy, combat thyroid-related metabolic slowdown, and get and stay fit for film shoots and photos, so exercise is a must!

Exercise is so important for those of us with hypothyroidism because it helps improve mood, sex drive, and sleep, reduces depression and anxiety, balances blood sugar, and helps control weight. Exercise is especially crucial for thyroid patients because it burns fat, helps the body release stored fat, and burns that stored fat for energy. It also really helps the overall hormone balance and reduces leptin and insulin resistance.

Exercise doesn't have to be intense—just low-intensity exercise, like a brisk thirty-minute walk—substantially helps balance these hormones, increases fat burning, and lowers insulin levels.

If you're walking outside or on a treadmill, one way to get the most out of it is to incorporate intervals. That's where you periodically build in a minute or two going at your maximum intensity, and then return to your regular pace. This really helps ramp up your metabolism, burn fat, and increase your endurance, without exhausting you.

Throw in some weight training, or weight-bearing exercise, and it's even better, because weight-bearing exercises improve muscle mass, and, here's the best part: muscle increases metabolism! The more muscle you have, the more calories you burn even at rest.

And finally, exercise improves lymphatic function. I didn't know much about the whole lymphatic issue before I developed a thyroid problem, but it's very important, especially for thyroid patients. When we don't move, the lymphatic system is unable to operate, and it can get clogged, backed up, and sluggish, which can cause bloating, swelling, water weight, fatigue, and poor immune function. The purpose of the lymphatic system is to absorb excess fluid, fat, toxins, and waste products; filter it all out; and return the filtered liquid—known as lymph—to the bloodstream. So, what about all that bloating and puffiness we have when we're hypothyroid? The answer is lymphatic exercise!

The only way to get the lymphatic system working is to "pump it out." That means walking, skipping rope, or, if you have a mini-trampoline, rebounder, or a backyard trampoline, gentle bouncing is a great lymphatic exercise. The T-Tapp program of DVDs from Teresa Tapp is also especially designed to be lymphatic, so it's a great option as well.

T-Tapp is Mary's favorite exercise program. (Despite the name, it has nothing to do with tap-dancing!) T-Tapp is a sequence of simple but very effective movements that cinch in muscles, help eliminate toxins, and build longer, leaner, denser muscle without bulk. The first week Mary did T-Tapp, she did three 40-minute sessions and lost twelve inches. It wasn't hard for her to decide to keep T-Tapping!

Beyond the benefits for weight and metabolism for thyroid patients, regular movement has so many incredible health benefits for us. Exercise is good for the heart and cholesterol levels. Getting the heart pumping makes it stronger and healthier, and it helps reduce the risk of cardiovascular disease and stroke.

In the end, it doesn't matter what you do—but find something that you like to do, because you'll need to be motivated to do it regularly. Whether it's walking, swimming, gardening, dancing, yoga, or a DVD like T-Tapp, make sure you are active every day.

Reasons to Move Every Day

Balance

Strength

Improved mood

Less depression

Reduced anxiety

Better sleep

More energy, less fatigue

Weight control, less weight gain

Helping redistribute weight that shifts due to hormones

Fewer body aches

Better bone density

Better heart health

Reduced number, intensity, and/or duration of hot flashes and
   night sweats in women over forty

Fun

Better sex drive!

Better sex!

One of the things I recommend, if you can afford it, is to work with a trainer. Even one or two sessions to get you started can help. I knew the fundamentals of fitness, but by working out with a trainer, I learned how to get the most out of my exercise and how to incorporate different muscles and routines, things I would never have thought of doing, such as intervals—short periods of getting the heart rate up, and then back down, to help raise metabolism and burn fat.

We all know we have to exercise. The real issue is, how do we get motivated? Here are some things that have been a help to me.

- Exercise with a friend—it really does help the time pass more quickly!
- Exercise earlier in the day—if I get in a workout early in the day, I feel so much better.
- Schedule your exercise on your calendar or PDA—I block out time to exercise onto my iPhone so that I know it's on the calendar!
- Take advantage of gyms at your workplace—some of my friends have nicely equipped gyms at their office, and they sometimes go in earlier in the morning, or do a workout during lunch or after work.
- Entertain yourself—listen to music or audiobooks or watch TV or movies while exercising. (This is one of my favorites!)
- Get a dog—Hank the Tank, our bulldog, doesn't move too quickly, but he still gets me out and moving!
- Fit fitness in—you've heard all of these, but it's worth repeating. Park farther away at the mall, take the stairs at the office, or go for a walk at lunch. Every little bit adds up.

Above all, don't use thyroid problems as an excuse not to exercise, unless your doctor has told you specifically that you can't! I know there are days when you won't have the energy to exercise—I've had many of them myself. But even then, take a gentle walk, or stretch—do something to keep moving.

I mentioned T-Tapp earlier, and Mary and I both highly recommend the work of our friend, exercise physiologist Teresa Tapp, who has wonderful fitness DVDs featuring her T-Tapp program of body-mind-muscle activation that you can do at home, no matter what your weight or fitness level. She's also developed special SneakyFit programs to "fit in fitness" into everyday activities, even sitting at your desk. We love them!

One thing to keep in mind is that you should not do too much exercise. (I know, not a problem for most of us!) If you push too hard, you may create inflammation, stress, raise cortisol, exhaust adrenals, and worsen your hormone imbalances. You'll know you're overexercising if you feel exhausted or need a nap after exercise, you feel sick or fluish after exercising, you have excessive pain in the day or two after exercise, or you feel exhausted and sluggish in the hours or days after your workout.

Other Exercise Tips

Here's a tip from Dr. Ron Rosedale, author of *The Rosedale Diet*: after dinner, do some mild resistance exercise or take a fifteen- to twenty-minute walk, ideally uphill. Since dinner is often our biggest meal of the day, planning some sort of physical activity after dinner may take advantage of the increase in metabolism after eating and help kickstart nighttime fat burning.

Another tip from Dr. Rosedale: if you do eat something high in sugar or processed carbohydrates, "exercise it off." He says, "If you don't burn off those starchy calories right away, they will raise your blood sugar, raise your leptin and insulin levels, prevent fat burning, and turn to fat, all of which get you right back to a deranged metabolism."

Teresa Tapp's T-Tapp Hoe-Downs are examples of a perfect exercise you can do right after eating. Just a few minutes of Hoe-Downs have been shown to measurably reduce blood sugar.

A FINAL NOTE

Mary has a whole book dedicated to the subject of weight loss and fitness for thyroid patients, and if you want to really delve into all the specifics, I highly recommend you read *The Thyroid Diet Revolution*.

If you are looking for a specific diet program, some of the books that thyroid patients have found helpful include:

Dr. Ann Louise Gittleman's *The Fat Flush Plan*
Dr. Ron Rosedale's *The Rosedale Diet*
Mark Sisson's *The Primal Blueprint*
Dr. Mark Hyman's *Ultrametabolism*
Dr. Arthur Agatston's *The South Beach Diet*

9

The Lazy Girl's Guide to Beauty

Everything has its beauty but not everyone sees it.
—CONFUCIUS

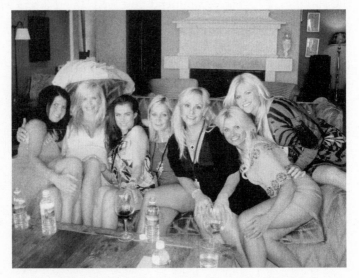

From left: *Kim, Gena (eight months pregnant), Alicia (my first roommate in L.A.), Janell, Sheila (my sister), Becky, and Jenn*

Every woman can be beautiful, and we all have the ability to look our best, even though we may face extra challenges—like the skin and hair issues that are so common for those of us with thyroid problems.

I thought it might be useful to talk about some of the beauty problems thyroid patients face, and about some solutions that help. Along the way, we'll share some of our favorite tips and products, and thyroid patients from our community will share their ideas as well.

KEEP IT SIMPLE

When you're tired and on the go, the last thing you need is a lengthy, complicated beauty routine.

People see photos of me in magazines, or see me on reruns of *Baywatch*, and they don't realize how much time went in to making me look that way. While working on *Baywatch* and *Sheena*, I was up at 3:30 or 4:00 a.m. so that I had time to shower and head to the set. Then it was several hours in the chair, getting my hair done and makeup applied, and all that was before I even set foot in front of the cameras! You are seeing the result of hours in the hair and makeup chair. I do NOT wake up looking like that!

This is why now that I'm a wife and mother, and often struggling to keep my energy up as a thyroid patient, I like to keep my routine as simple as possible. I wash my face, put on some moisturizer with SPF—I've already spent too much time in the sun running up and down that beach!—put my hair in a ponytail, and I'm ready to go.

But one important note: ALWAYS TAKE OFF YOUR MAKEUP! Since I was a teenager, even if I'm drop-dead tired after a long day, I've been religious about washing off my makeup before I go to bed. Always clean your face, because going to bed with makeup worsens puffiness, clogs and enlarges your pores, and makes skin look dull and lifeless.

EYE PUFFINESS

One common hypothyroidism side effect is puffiness and bagginess around the eyes—under the eyes, the eyelids, and under the eyebrows. When I had a morning shoot and noticed that I was especially puffy, I would cut cold cucumbers, and place the slices over my eyes. I also always kept tea bags in the refrigerator. Let them steep a bit the night before, take them out of the water, and refrigerate. Then place the cold tea bag on your eye to help reduce puffiness. Nothing fancy . . . plain, inexpensive generic store-brand black tea seems to work best.

Some other tips for puffy eyes:

- Some people like to keep teaspoons in the refrigerator . . . and when your eyes are puffy, put a cold spoon—curved side down—on each eye to help reduce puffiness.
- If you're in a rush, after you've washed your face or had a shower in the morning, rinse a few times with very cold water. The cold shrinks blood vessels and can reduce puffiness.
- Stay hydrated. If you're not getting enough water, your eye area may puff up.
- Cover eyes with cool water on a damp cloth or paper for a few moments, followed by a gentle massage.
- Keep your head elevated while sleeping. This can help minimize puffiness in the morning.
- Watch your salt intake.

One member of our thyroid community, Yvette, swears by MAC's Fast Response Eye Cream to bring down puffiness, and another member, Mara, loves Benefit's Ooh La Lift.

DRY SKIN

Dry skin is one of the most common skin and beauty complaints among thyroid patients. I naturally have dry skin, and my thyroid problem hasn't helped. Now that I'm in my forties, I want to take particular care of my skin to minimize wrinkles and fine lines.

My favorite skin care product is the Ole Henriksen Micro/ Mini Peel System, a three-step process that includes a scrub, a serum, and a calming cream. I do this at least every week to keep my skin in good shape.

I also use Peter Thomas Roth facial cleansers morning and night, and I always moisturize afterward. My favorite is Kiehl's facial moisturizer; they have a regular version for night and one with sun protection for the daytime. (Speaking of which—never go out without sunscreen on your face! It's a key to keeping young-looking skin!)

Mary and I are both fans of a relatively new product called NeriumAD. Derived from an extract of the oleander plant, it dramatically improves fine lines, crow's-feet, frown lines, and marionette lines, as well as tightening pores and improving skin texture. In Mary's case, she eliminated two deep vertical frown lines, and a deep horizontal forehead line in less than two months. For me, just a few days, and my skin tightened up amazingly. Who needs Botox?

The most popular moisturizer by far according to our thyroid community members is the CeraVe lotions and creams, which are not expensive and available at drugstores. They were frequently mentioned as being especially effective for dryness all over the body, including the feet. Coconut oil used externally is also popular with thyroid patients.

Some other dry skin tips:

- "Especially in the winter, I don't use very hot water when I shower. When I turn off the water, I grab the baby oil and apply it all over while I'm still wet. Do not rinse, just towel off. Then I use Bath & Body Works body butter. I don't have dry or itchy skin, and it stays soft all day and night. It's the best way to combat my dry skin!"—Michelle
- "I'm in the beauty business, and I recommend a daily gentle exfoliation for face and body followed by an oil-based moisturizer to keep skin more hydrated."—Angie
- "I like Paula's Choice 2% BHA Gel Exfoliant for getting rid of flaky dry skin and controlling acne at the same time."—Anne
- "I use baby oil . . . it's really good for dry face skin . . . just a few drops before getting out of the shower."—Andrew
- "When my skin gets superdry I use olive oil on my face and body a few minutes before jumping in the shower. It might be a little messy, but it works for me."—Elizabeth
- "I am a nurse so dry hands and eczema are a constant battle. Lately I have had good luck with Vaseline petroleum jelly with cocoa butter at night."—Mary Beth

Dry lips are also a common problem.

- "For lips, I use Carmex. I've been using this at bedtime for twenty-five years and I always wake up with moisturized lips."—Ellen
- "I sleep with Blistex on my lips and it's on all day."—Lee-anne

Many thyroid patients complain about having dry, cracked feet. Some of the favorite tips for dealing with this problem include the following:

- "I use organic coconut oil, and it does wonders for my dry, cracked feet."—Lisa
- "I use the Neutrogena intensive moisturizer, and then wear socks to bed. Really helps my feet."—Cathi
- "For aching, puffy feet, I rub some Badger Headache Soother (smells great!) on my feet and put socks on. I leave it on overnight, if possible."—Lauren

THIN OR MISSING BROWS

Eyebrows can be an adventure for thyroid patients, and one thing I've learned along the way is that loss of the hair in the outer edge of the eyebrow is a classic sign of hypothyroidism. On his television show, Dr. Mehmet Oz has demonstrated how to take a pencil, hold it straight up next to the outside of your lip, and if the outer edge of your eyebrow doesn't meet the pencil, that could be a sign you're hypothyroid. Who knew?

My eyebrows are already light in color, and with the thyroid issues, there have been times when they get really sparse. For daytime, I particularly like Anastasia Beverly Hills Brow Gel (it comes clear or tinted). You just brush it on and go. For evening events or work, I have a Sephora eyebrow kit that I love, which thickens the brows and fills them in a bit.

A number of thyroid patients have told us that they've had their eyebrows cosmetically tattooed. This permanently adds some visual "fill" to eyebrows. But make sure that you get it done by a professional.

Some other ideas from the thyroid patient community:

- "I was introduced to eyebrow threading a number of years ago and haven't looked back. It helps keep them shaped, and makes them look thicker."—Elizabeth
- "A makeup artist told me to just put a bit of dark brown eyeshadow along my brow to fill in the gaps. It works pretty well, but fortunately my eyebrows have started growing back now that I'm on thyroid treatment."—Anne
- "The new eyebrow markers by Laura Geller and by NYC Cosmetics are awesome—you can draw wisps that are like eyebrow hairs so that missing outer third is far less noticeable!"—Lisa
- "I go to the Brow Bar at Benefit Cosmetics to get my brows done and they've shaped them so that they look fuller."—Mara
- "For eyebrows, I use an eyebrow pencil the same color as my brows, and fill them in, and extend the brow line a little."—Michele
- "I love Anastasia Beverly Hills Brow Powder Duo, I've used it for years! It's $20, but will last a year at least." —Rebecca

Several also recommended the bareMinerals Brow Color (a powder), including Kathy, who said, "It works great and looks natural if the salesperson helps you pick the right color!"

SPARSE EYELASHES

I have trouble with my lashes—they are never thick enough, and have been especially thin since my thyroid condition developed.

You can try Latisse, a prescription medication that thickens eyelashes. This medication did work for me. But to be honest, I started to worry that it might change my eye color—it can sometimes affect eye color as a side effect—and so I stopped using it.

Mary swears by RapidLash Eyelash & Eyebrow Enhancing Serum. It's available at beauty supply stores and online. She has said that it really thickened her lashes, but you have to give it about four weeks before you really start to see a difference.

I'm also a firm believer in false eyelashes. I use them all the time, especially if I'm going out at night. I don't have a favorite brand here—I find the drugstore has the best false lashes. If I'm going for a daytime natural look, I'll use thinner ones, but if it's a nighttime event, I go for a thicker, full lash. The key is to make sure when you peel it off that it fits your eye. You may need to trim the width and length a bit, then put a little bit of glue on the line, and the trick for me is to let it kind of sit for a minute, blow on it, make the glue tacky, then apply. Keep the false lash as close as you can to your natural eyelash line. Always start with a coat of mascara before you apply the lashes, and after you apply, add another coat of mascara, and you're good to go. It's a good idea to practice with the lashes to make sure they fit before you try them for a special event.

Some other lash tips from the thyroid community:

- "I always use an eyelash curler first, before I apply mascara. It makes my eyelashes look longer, it makes my eyes appear more open and I just feel like I look fresher."—Lisa

- "I LOVE Benefit's They're Real! mascara."—Mara
- "I get permanent eyelashes applied . . . they last about seven weeks . . . when energy stays low it is so much better to wash face, moisturize, apply lipstick, and GO!"—Alicia

HAIR CHALLENGES

Hair issues are one of the biggest beauty challenges for thyroid patients. Hypothyroidism can make your hair shed rapidly and change in texture, becoming coarse, dry, tangly, or hard to manage.

So many thyroid patients at our communities complain about their hair, and holy Hannah, can I relate!

When I became hypothyroid, and my symptoms were coming on at 100 miles an hour, one of the first things I noticed was my hair. It became very brittle, and looked like someone had taken a cigarette lighter and singed the edges. I have medium-thick, not superfine, hair and I usually have a decent head of hair. Then it started falling out. But suddenly, I was wondering what to do with my hair, and trying new conditioners and so on to try to get some body.

Mary has had the same problem. She has long, usually thick hair, but at one point, she had lost so much hair due to thyroid problems that if you pulled it all together into a ponytail, it had the thickness of a pencil! One doctor told her she was just stressed out . . . that was why she was losing her hair. Apparently, Mary told the doctor, "You bet I'm stressed out! I'm stressed out because I'm losing my hair!"

Even after treatment, my hair is still somewhat coarse, and shedding more than I'd like. But I'm taking vitamins, supplements, and iron, and doing my best, and it's coming around.

Because I have extremely dry hair, and even more with my thyroid condition, I try hard to keep it moisturized. I like the various products that contain Moroccan argan oil. For shampoos and conditioners, I don't need anything especially fancy. I like Pantene, Kerastase, and Aveeno products.

Mary is a fan of Pantene's Breakage Defense line. When hair gets tangled or coarse, she has found that this product definitely reduces the breakage, and helps hair stay smoother and less tangled.

We both color our hair. One tip—don't be afraid to dye your own hair. Believe it or not, I've colored my own hair since I was sixteen, and I will color my hair until the end! I use L'Oréal—usually a shade of natural or golden blond—and I touch it up every three weeks or so.

The thyroid community shares their dry hair suggestions:

- "I try not to blow-dry my hair unless I absolutely have to. I live in a cold climate so in the winter it's harder. I try to give my hair a break. I also use a natural bristle brush, which adds shine, as well as Moroccan oil products to help control frizz."—Elizabeth
- "My hair is superdry so I swear by shampoos and conditioners with argan oil!"—Kristen
- "I use Wen for my hair—no sulfates or anything. And let my hair dry as much as possible before I use a dryer. I also use a spritz of argan oil before I straighten my hair."—Leeanne

- "I use ayurvedic amla oil for my hair. I rub in a teaspoon one hour before washing, or even leave it in all night and shampoo in the morning."—Pat
- "Pureology's Hydrate Shine Max keeps my frizzies and dryness at bay. You only need a little bit. I saturate the ends of my hair with it to prevent breakage."—Joy
- "I have tried a lot of hair products and have had good results with It's a 10 Miracle Leave-In Product."—Judy
- "I do a coconut oil treatment for an hour before washing my hair, and Moroccan argan oil to help control the frizz!!"—Natalie

Thyroid patients also have a number of tips and tricks for thinning hair.

- "I use hair-thickening and hair-volumizing products to give the illusion of thicker, fuller hair, since I've lost about 40 percent of my hair since the thyroid surgery."—Hanne
- "I love Nioxin shampoo and conditioner for hair loss." —Cass
- "I get my bangs cut more layery in the front to help disguise some hair loss I have there."—Lisa
- "For thinning hair, I use a curling iron to give it some lift, and spritz with a little hairspray."—Michele
- "I just started using a natural bristle brush a few months ago and I love it!! It is more gentle, and my hair has less breakage."—Kim
- "I'm taking 5,000 mcg of biotin daily, that keeps my hair healthy and strong."—Lavonne

Hair Extensions and Clip-ins

I sometimes have to have extensions in my hair, because I still haven't gotten back to a place where I'm fully satisfied with my hair volume.

There have also been times with my thyroid problem when my hair was horribly thin, so bad that even a ponytail didn't work, and I didn't want permanent extensions. So I turned to these gorgeous clip-in hair pieces from Jessica Simpson. It's a fun look for under $100, and they're easy to use. You can clip on an entire ponytail, or if you're wearing your hair down, you take little sections where the clip will be, go underneath the layers, tease and rat it up a little, clip it in to anchor, and shazam, you have a full head of hair! Gives you that extra oomph, and it really makes you feel good about yourself.

Celebrity hairstylist Tabatha Coffey also has a new line of clip-in extensions called Luxhair How that look great.

Mary likes the little stretchy poufs of fake hair they sell at the drugstore, and usually they're less than $15. She said when her hair was thinning, she would pull it back into a bun, and pop one of those over it to hide her skimpy little ponytail, and it got her through until her hair grew back in. Whew!

Celebrity hairstylist Brent Hardgrave, who works with a number of thyroid patients, recommends a new type of salon-applied human hair extensions called Simplicity. They are fast and easy to apply (it usually takes no more than an hour), and since they are not glued to hair shafts, they don't cause "traction alopecia"—a condition that can be caused by regular hair extensions and result in your losing even more hair. They also don't pull on the scalp and cause pain or tension headaches. They are only available through trained stylists. But Mary watched Brent transform a girl with very thin, flat hair into someone with so much thick, shiny hair that she could be in a shampoo commercial, in about thirty minutes, and the final look was so natural you wouldn't know it wasn't her own hair. It's expensive, but it may be an option for thyroid patients who want hair to look great for a special occasion.

Understanding Thyroid-Related Hair Loss

Hair is truly a barometer of health, because hair cells are some of the fastest growing in the body, and so they reflect what's going on in terms of health, nutrition, and hormones. When the body is in crisis, redirecting energy elsewhere, hair cells can shut down, and that means hair loss. Situations that can cause hair loss include hormonal changes, poor diet and nutritional deficiencies, a variety of medications, surgery, and many medical conditions—notably, thyroid disease.

When you have a thyroid problem, or when you hit your forties, the most common type of hair loss is androgenetic alopecia, also known as female-pattern hair loss. What happens is that hormone imbalances cause testosterone to more easily metabolize to dihydrotestosterone (DHT), which then causes the hair follicles to reduce in size, interrupting hair growth. Hair texture, diameter, and length change, the growth cycles get shorter, and individual hair shafts can get shorter and thinner until no hair growth is evident at all.

Many people notice rapid hair loss as a symptom of hypothyroidism. Some say this is the most troublesome symptom of their thyroid problem—the thinning hair or drains clogged with lost hair, often accompanied by changes in texture so that it is dry, coarse, and tangled. Interestingly, some people have actually told us that their thyroid problems were first discovered by their hairdressers!

Proper thyroid treatment can help some cases of hormonally driven hair loss. If you're experiencing hair loss and are just starting thyroid treatment, it's likely that the loss will slow down, and eventually stop, once levels are balanced. This may take a few months. But don't panic. Most people don't go bald! Mary estimates that at one point, she lost almost half of her long, thick hair. But over time, and with proper thyroid treatment, it eventually did get back to normal.

If you continue to lose hair, you need to make sure that it's not your particular type of thyroid hormone replacement. Prolonged or excessive hair loss is a side effect of levothyroxine drugs (like Synthroid and Levoxyl) in some people. Many of us don't know this, and our doctors don't either. Both Mary and I noticed far less hair loss once we switched from levothyroxine drugs to natural desiccated thyroid drugs, like Armour Thyroid and Nature-Throid.

Mary is a fan of evening primrose oil—about 1,300 to 1,500 mg a day—as well as the recommended daily dosage of Cooper Complete Dermatologic Health (Hair, Skin & Nail) formula, to help counteract periods of hair loss. The combination of supplements not only slows down her hair loss but stops it after about two months, and new hair starts to grow back (watch the hairline for small baby hairs regrowing), and the new hair is normal, not coarse or tangly.

Some other ways to help with hair loss include the following:

- Finasteride (Propecia): This drug is available by prescription. It's not for women of child-bearing years, but it can help postmenopausal women with hair loss.
- Minoxidil (Rogaine, Keranique): This over-the-counter drug, which comes in a topical solution, may slow down hair loss, or help maintain the hair on the head, and in some people, it may also help trigger hair regrowth after several months.
- Corticosteroids—"steroid" drugs, usually injected into the patchy spots, taken orally or administered topically as an ointment or cream.
- The HairMax LaserComb: This is the only FDA-approved consumer device to treat hair loss. It's expensive, usually around $500, and the results are mixed, but some people swear by it.
- Iron supplements: Make sure you have your blood levels of ferritin checked by your doctor or a self-testing lab. If the levels are below 80 (on a scale of around 20 to 100), your hair loss may be at least in part related to your ferritin levels, and supplemental iron may help. But always make sure you take any iron supplements at least three to four hours apart from any thyroid medications.

In addition to evening primrose oil and iron, some other natural approaches that are helpful for hair loss include:

B-complex vitamins
DHEA
Green tea
Lysine

L-arginine

Methylsulfonylmethane (MSM)

Saw palmetto

Pygeum (*Prunus africana*)/beta-sitosterol

Zinc

MAKEUP IDEAS

One of the complaints from thyroid patients is that our skin can frequently look dull or lifeless, or even patchy and discolored at times. This is where makeup comes in.

You don't need to spend a lot on makeup—some of my favorites come from the regular drugstore. You also don't have to pick one line; I tend to mix and match my favorite cosmetics. In fact, you probably find that different products from different lines are really your best bet.

To even out and liven up my skin tone, I live by L'Oréal True Match compact makeup, a creamy foundation that's good for my dry skin.

Mary, whose skin is oilier and prone to breakouts, loves the Bare Escentuals powder foundations. These tend to be popular with other thyroid patients because they have few allergens and don't tend to irritate sensitive skin. Mary also swears by a makeup primer—and loves Revlon's PhotoReady Perfecting Primer—which helps makeup go on more smoothly and keeps her skin from getting too oily.

If you have discolorations, or vitiligo, a number of thyroid patients mentioned that they've had good luck with Dermablend makeup, which helps cover imperfections and vitiligo patches.

A member of our thyroid community, Angie, is in the beauty business, and she says, "Blush with highlighter really perks up a tired face—apply from apples up to temples." Angie's right!

My favorite blush? Hands down, it's NARS Orgasm Blush—it gives you a little bit of frost and a light natural color. NARS also has a highlighter—Super Orgasm Illuminator—it's a gel that comes in a container, and after you squeeze out a little dot, it gives you a dewy glow on the apple of your cheek that may be missing when you're dragging around with dry skin and thyroid-related fatigue. It's a great boost when you are looking pale or tired. I've gotten Mary totally hooked on the NARS blush and illuminator as well!

FASHION FOR THYROID PATIENTS

It's not just how you look but what you wear. But you don't need all sorts of designer outfits—I don't! I'm a fan of Target myself.

But if there is one thing I can suggest to every female thyroid patient reading this book: invest in a few pairs of Spanx! I can't live without Spanx undergarments; they are the best clothing item ever made! You can get body shapers, tummy trimmers, and long, full-body shapers with legs that are almost like a tank dress. I have a couple of different Spanx options to put under dresses and shirts. They help tighten everything up, make short work of that muffin top, and give you a nice, clean line.

My other advice is to invest in a great pair of black pants. For those of us who need some tummy control, there are some great styles that have slimming panels built inside the pants. Shape FX have some great shapewear pants with slimming panels. And Mary swears by the Victoria's Secret VS Siren straight-leg jeans that have some stretch in them. You get a stylish slim fit, with a little bit of stretch for the hypothyroid figure or for those days when you're feeling bloated.

I always have a few tops that are looser around the bottom. They are great to camouflage muffin top, or to wear on those days when thyroid bloat is particularly evident.

And don't forget hats. If your hair is thinning, there are some stylish hats and great woolly caps that can look adorable and help hide thinning hair on days when you just don't feel like doing much to your hair.

TAKE TIME OUT FOR BEAUTY

When you're struggling to feel and look well with your thyroid condition, don't shortchange yourself. Make some time just for you.

As a wife and mother, it's not often I have a few minutes to myself. But I do try to schedule time to get some exercise, shop for healthy foods, eat right, and enjoy the occasional pampering session. It's so important. I know how easy it is to put yourself last on the to-do list, but that really does shortchange everyone around you in the end.

When I'm going out to do something special, for example, I like to have a special routine, to carve out a bit of space. I put on some music, take a relaxing bath, put in some hot rollers, and spend a bit of time doing my makeup—usually around fifteen minutes or so. It's setting a mood for myself and taking time out, regardless of how busy I am.

(One piece of advice, though—if you have little ones like I

do, make sure you have a lock on the bathroom door! There's nothing like Mommy taking a bath to inspire children to barge in! I love my children, but we all need a few minutes of time to ourselves, right?)

And it may be the most important thing of all, and it's something I have to work on, too. But it's really important to be kind and compassionate—to yourself. And that starts with what you say to yourself, about yourself. Don't ever say anything to yourself that you wouldn't be willing to say to your best friend, or your child. So stop the "I look fat in this!" And the "my hair is awful," or "I have suitcases under my eyes" nonsense. You would never say that to your best girlfriends, so don't say it to yourself. Be your own champion! Appreciate your good qualities, your best features . . . celebrate them!

My young daughter and I have a ritual. Every night after her bath, we look in the mirror and say together, "I am a strong, confident, beautiful girl." That's something we've done since she was six months old—I want her to grow up feeling good about herself, fighting for her rights and being strong in her beliefs, with boundaries in place. I want her to have fun, give love, and be loved, but to have the boundaries a woman should have.

So the next time you look at yourself in the mirror, say, "I am a strong, confident, beautiful—and yes, sexy—woman!" And make sure it's loud enough so we all can hear you!

10

Finding Our Life Preservers

Hope is patience with the lamp lit.

—TERTULLIAN

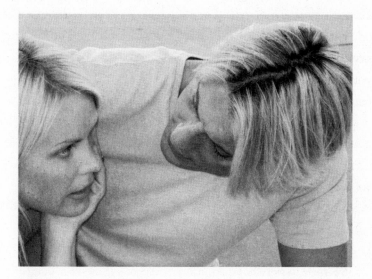

I've shared so much about my own health experiences, life, love, and motherhood, but as I look back, there are some things that have been a help to both Mary and me that we hope will also be a help to you in living a happy, healthy life with your thyroid condition.

Since I played a lifeguard, let's call them our life preservers!

APPRECIATING THE SUPPORTIVE
AND HELPFUL PEOPLE IN YOUR LIFE

Whether it's a friend, family member, or spouse, be sure to openly and vocally appreciate the people who are supportive and who help you, especially through the tougher times.

For me, the key person is my husband, Cale. He's a glass-half-full kind of guy, and when I get stressed or overworried, he's always been the voice of reason, bringing me back down to earth. It wasn't always like that, though, because in the beginning, Cale didn't really understand how hard it was for me, and he has readily admitted it:

> As an athlete, I'm used to a "suck it up" mentality. In sports, there's a difference between being injured and something hurting. If something hurts, you just "suck it up" and play. So that was my initial reaction—at first I thought Gena should just suck it up.
>
> But I quickly saw how much she was suffering and struggling. There were days when it was hard enough for her to simply get out of bed, much less function. I would feel horrible if I were in her shoes, so in my perspective, the best thing I could do was to help pick up the slack and be as supportive as possible.

Because I am married to one of the truly good guys, he has worked to really understand and be compassionate. When you find people like this in your life, hang on to them, and let them know how you appreciate them!

I hear stories from other thyroid patients about unsympathetic partners or spouses, and it brings tears to my eyes. But it makes Cale mad!

> I am disgusted when I hear about unsympathetic husbands or partners. To be honest, I feel like the men who treat the women in their lives horribly should have the experience of thyroid disease firsthand themselves . . . then they might understand.
>
> And seriously, if I was sitting there and some guy was talking about his wife or girlfriend being unattractive, or fat, or lazy, because she had thyroid disease, I'd think I'd be so fed up I might lean across the table and knock the guy out!

He wouldn't really do that, but it's a great feeling to know he's got my back! Make sure that you appreciate the people in your life who have your back.

Surrounding Yourself with Optimists

I have a tendency to be a bit of a glass-half-empty girl. I tend to be a worrier, and assume the worst sometimes, so I value optimism and positivity in others. It's one thing I constantly work on in myself. I try to meditate, to work on a positive attitude, and try to really see things more optimistically.

But I've got good sense—and in Cale, I found a true optimist. It's one of his best qualities. Cale always looks on the bright side. That doesn't mean he downplays legitimate concerns, but he's always looking for a positive way forward toward our goals. (Makes sense as a hockey player!)

Despite her own health challenges, my friend Janell has always been optimistic and positive as well. I try to learn from these wonderful optimists in my life.

246 BEAUTIFUL INSIDE AND OUT

Janell always tells me to believe in myself, and that's something that really rings true to me. She always tells me, "You can handle this, you can do this." Regardless of what the challenge is, she always gives me the pep talk that every girlfriend needs, which gives me a little spring in my step and gets me back where I need to be. It's those times when you're tired, down, defeated, can't remember anything, don't feel good, are trying to raise children, feeling exhausted, and thinking, "How am I going to do this?" And then I hear that little voice, and it sounds like Janell, saying, "You can do this!"

Having a chronic disease is enough of a challenge that you don't need people around you who drag you down further. So, when taking time to be with friends and family, making new friends, or choosing a partner, my advice: focus on the optimistic people in your life!

A SPECIAL NOTE TO
PARTNERS AND SPOUSES

Cale was willing to share some thoughts about being the partner of someone with a chronic illness, and I think his ideas are worth sharing.

> With Gena, I made the commitment, and we're a team. Whatever it takes to get through, we'll do. So my advice, first of all, is to be understanding. Really dig down deep and try to understand your partner's feelings. You have to imagine what it would feel like if you were the one diagnosed with a disease, having days when you can't get out of bed, or can't do what you feel needs to be done for your family.

I also think it's essential to develop compassion. Honestly, I don't understand how someone can not be compassionate about someone they love. Because to me, the hardest part of all of this is knowing what Gena is going through.

It's also so important to love the woman, not the image. I'm lucky to have married a woman who is naturally beautiful. But Gena has had times—when she gained weight, or lost hair, or was puffy—when she felt far from beautiful, even though others might not agree. Especially coming from a business where she's had to focus on her looks for half of her life, and where people are always judging her, it's hard for her not to judge herself harshly. And she's always the one who is hardest on herself. But I've never thought that she didn't look amazing. She always looks like Gena to me. I'm so in love with her it doesn't matter. And above all, I love what's inside, her heart, her spirit, her compassion.

I told you I found a good one!

JOINING A SUPPORT COMMUNITY/ DON'T SUFFER IN SILENCE

As I mentioned, one of the most eye-opening parts of my journey was when I finally found a community of thyroid patients. There I finally was able to learn, to share my own story, to vent to like-minded people who understood exactly what I was going through.

I know that it can be hard to think about opening yourself up to people you don't know, but joining a support group—whether an online thyroid group, a group for chronic diseases, or a local, in-person support group—is a crucial part of the healing process.

This is one of the key reasons that both Mary and I have started thyroid communities on the web and Facebook.

On my Thyroid Sexy Facebook page, one of the group's most articulate members is Linda Adams, a Hashimoto's patient from Florida. Like me, Linda was misdiagnosed for years. Linda is smart and compassionate, and I invited her to help out on the Thyroid Sexy page, and Linda graciously agreed and has been so supportive of what I was trying to do. Here's what she has said: "It's so important for people with this illness to have the support of family and friends. But it is equally important to have a place to come to, to 'virtually vent' with others who are facing the same trials and tribulations, a safe place that offers hope to people when they feel there is no hope left. It encourages everyone to keep fighting, to keep trying to find the right doctor and the right treatment."

There are many different support communities, many of them online, so you can even remain anonymous. But I promise you . . . join one, share your story, lend your ear to others, and you will make new friends for life. And, unlike family and friends, a good support community never tires of talking about thyroid disease!

Stephanie is a member of both of our groups: "Mary and Gena have been my salvation. The support I get is overwhelming and I feel nothing but gratitude. I am a huge thyroid advocate now. I never shut up about it and they have empowered me to reach out to others and let them know that they are not alone."

Jacqueline has also found Mary's group helpful:

I learned a tremendous amount from Mary about the disease and the people behind thyroid disorders. Her story is inspiring because she went from patient to advocate through thorough research and not settling for quick answers. As an RN, I am in awe of the amount of time and energy Mary puts into educating herself and others. For myself, I changed the way I view my health and the choices I make. I'm never done learning about my condition and I deserve good support.

Katarina loves Gena's Facebook page:

I am really grateful to have someone who knows how terrible it feels to have this disease. No one in my life (other than my therapist and my mother) understands how miserable thyroid diseases make you. I love that Gena is out there supporting us through our battles and caring about everyone.

BEING ON THE LOOKOUT FOR THYROID PROBLEMS IN YOUR CHILDREN

For those of us with autoimmune thyroid disease, we need to be aware that our children are also at higher risk of developing thyroid conditions.

I've made sure that my autoimmune Hashimoto's disease is in my children's medical history. And Mary has made sure that her teenage daughter had a full thyroid panel done after she reached puberty.

This is another issue for our thyroid community.

Chris was in her early thirties when she was finally diagnosed, after years of symptoms.

My daughter developed an enlarged thyroid at the age of nine. I noticed it immediately, and her awesome pediatrician referred her to an equally awesome endocrinologist, who started her on levothyroxine with frequent blood draws and a goal of treating symptoms. At the initial visit, I told him my story and he told me that Hashimoto's tends to run in families. Now my daughter is twenty-one, and we both struggle with some continuing symptoms.

Crimson has had thyroid issues since she was ten: "My son was also recently diagnosed with a low thyroid. I am so happy I've been through it all, so I can help him on his journey as well."

NEVER GIVING UP

One of the things that all of us feel is crucial is that you don't give up. You are worth it. So even if it seems like you're spinning your wheels, you need to stick with it.

It took Denise, a member of our thyroid community, sixteen different doctors over four years to get her diagnosis.

I've been symptomatic since I was a teenager, always freezing, and experiencing depression and anxiety. I went to doctors back then, but they couldn't diagnose me. By the time I was in my twenties, I'd learned that my sister had Hashimoto's, and my mother, aunts, etc. all had thyroid issues. I even brought this up to my doctors about the strong family history, but nobody could diagnose me. By the time I hit my early thirties, things got so bad; I had muscle aches in my legs, chronic dry eyes, horrific fatigue—not just feeling sleepy, but bone-crushing fatigue like being hit by a truck!—brain fog, inability to concentrate, dry skin, hair falling out in clumps, tingling and numbness in the extremities, and heart palpitations. I would go to my doctors, telling them I think I was pretty sure it was hypothyroidism, and all of them just ran a TSH test and said "your TSH is fine, you're not overweight, you can't be hypothyroid, you're fine."

After sixteen doctors, I finally found an integrative doctor who ran free T3, free T4, thyroid antibodies, and reverse T3. It turns out my free T3 was in the gutter, and he said just from listening to my symptoms he'd have diagnosed me with hypothyroidism.

I want everybody to know there is help. You have to find the right doctor. If your doctor is only testing TSH, you need a new doctor. I went to sixteen doctors, and from my experience, the integrative doctors are the ones who seem to have a clue. Don't give up the fight.

BEING YOUR OWN ADVOCATE/ DOING YOUR HOMEWORK

As Mary and I both learned, it's essential to learn, follow up, and stay on top of things health-wise. Being your own advocate is truly one of the most important changes you can make for your own health.

One of our thyroid community members, Renee, found out she had a thyroid nodule and Hashimoto's hypothyroidism a number of years ago only when she requested thyroid bloodwork after three miscarriages in a row. Says Renee:

The doctor told me to get the nodule checked every year. We then moved four times to four states, due to my husband being in the army. And along the way, it took work staying on top of my health with all the moves and new doctors. But it was worth it to be able to give birth to my two children. Plus, due to my follow-up, I learned last year that the nodule had become cancerous, and was able to get treated. I can't stress enough the importance of being your own advocate and reading all the info out there to educate yourself!

Ally had just turned twenty-two when she became extremely fatigued and overweight.

Physically, emotionally, and mentally I was a different person. The worst part was that I was a newlywed, and I had to put my husband through all that. I was diagnosed with Hashimoto's hypothyroidism. The first thing I did was educate myself. I found Mary's website, read all her books, and I was so relieved to find out there were others who went through what I went through. It's been four years, and it's still a daily battle. Everything happens for a reason, and I try to find the good in things. If the reason I have all these problems is so I can relate to others who have these problems, that's fine. Because I know when I was undiagnosed, I wished I could find someone who would understand, and I did. If I can be that light for someone else, that's a blessing. That's what thyroid awareness is all about.

Kristen, a thyroid patient, says, "The biggest thing I have learned is that educating yourself is the most powerful and best thing you can do for yourself. And when in doubt, ask questions!" Heidi has been a nurse for twenty years, but even she has found research important. "I thought I knew it all!! HA! I now know that I knew little about the endocrine system, and after reading so much about it in the past year, I still don't know all that there is to know! I have to say that if it wasn't for Gena's Facebook page, I might still be in the 'dark' about all this thyroid misinformation!"

AVOIDING DRAMA

The last thing we need as thyroid patients is drama, because drama causes stress, and that makes it much harder to feel well. One area where there can be so much drama is in dealing with blended families, but it's one area where my entire family has successfully refused to allow drama. My ex, Greg; my husband, Cale; and I all work hard to have a respectful and friendly relationship, and it works. And it helps that Spencer, Caia, Hudson, and Stella are wonderful children whom we all love very much.

Who better than my older son, Spencer, to share his thoughts?

With a divorce, people can get at each other's throats, and poison their kids with all their hostility and anger about the other parent. But that's not how it is in my family. My dad will come over and hang out with my little brother and sister, even babysit so my mom and Cale can go out. And Cale has been such a supportive member of my family. He's even coached my hockey teams. Our family is awesome.

I agree!

Do what you can to bypass drama in your life. Focus on creating stability, peace, and calm—these are all much more conducive to good health!

ACCEPT YOURSELF,
GIVE UP TRYING TO BE PERFECT

Being in the entertainment business, I lived for a long time with the expectation that I would be "perfect"—with perfect hair, perfect teeth, perfect skin, a perfect figure. It's an awful feeling, and you end up constantly feeling like you don't measure up. For those of us with thyroid issues, we can also have the expectation that we have to be perfect—perfect moms, perfect wives, perfect friends, perfect employees, and so on. It's a stress that makes you feel worse.

Sarah describes her experience:

> I have had a lot of internal battles. It was hard to keep weight off. I never felt beautiful. I'm this person who wants everything to be perfect, and that's not real life. So I pushed through. I don't let my diagnosis define me. Finally, about three years ago, I got on track, started working out, eating well, and I finally gained control . . . and balance. Through all the trials, I have only become stronger, and I hope that I can now inspire others . . . in their self-worth, and their abilities to do whatever they put their mind to. It's been a crazy journey, and it'll continue being a crazy journey. It's a day-by-day process, but I have accepted where I'm at now, and I'm so grateful. I am not the disease, and it's not me . . . it's part of me, but it does not define me.

COMMUNICATING AND FORGIVING

It is so essential to communicate. I've realized that keeping things inside is not always the healthiest thing you can do. I try to stay in touch with family, friends, and colleagues, and make time to really connect, find out how the people in my life are doing, be there for them, and share my own experiences and stories.

One of the most important people I've learned to communicate with is my mother.

We had our ups and downs through my teenage years, but motherhood truly gave me a new appreciation for my mother and the challenges she faced, raising three children on her own. Still, I had some leftover pain from the past, and over time, I've managed to say my piece to my mother, and it's been amazing. Sharing how I felt about our earlier life together transformed our relationship.

Now I accept my mother for who she is. I honor her and love her. She's a beautiful person. It was so important for me to learn that we all make mistakes, and instead of pointing the finger at my mother, I've come to recognize and understand what she was going through. As I've gotten older, walking in her shoes, I came to understand that she loved us, and she did what she had to do. I was really able to let go of a lot of pain.

I don't know if I'll ever find peace with my father, or have a relationship with him, but I haven't completely given up hope that it might happen one day. Miracles do happen.

But in the end, compassion and forgiveness go a long way toward health and happiness.

DON'T LISTEN TO THE HATERS

There are always going to be people who complain about you, criticize you, try to run you down, or turn positives into negatives. And it's my job to tell you, do NOT listen to them!

There are so many angry, sad, and disturbed individuals with too much time on their hands. In my case, there have always been reporters, paparazzi, nutty fans, fellow actors, and members of the media who have judged me—I didn't look this way, or that way, should have said this, or done that. They've critiqued everything from my acting to my clothing to my hairdo to the color of my nail polish, often right to my face! (Yes, I went through that harrowing experience known as a "Red Carpet Interview" with the infamous Joan Rivers, and I've lived to tell about it!)

These days, if you add in the anonymity of the Internet, where anyone can write pretty much anything they want about you, with no repercussions . . . well, let's just say that no matter what you do, someone out there will find a way to tear you down about it.

If I cured cancer, I have no doubt that someone would create a web page, Tweet, or post on Facebook that "Gena Lee Nolin didn't cure heart disease! Wow, what a loser!"

Mary and I have both been on the receiving end of more than our fair share of crazy stuff. And we both have had to learn that you get more done, and you're much happier and healthier, when you ignore people who want to bring you down.

That's why I encourage you to just close out the negative people in your life. I once saw a great poster that I loved. It said, "Don't let the negative people take up valuable real estate in your head!"

Don't listen to the obnoxious people talking about you behind your back in the grocery line or saying things right to your face.

Don't go back to a doctor who talks to you disrespectfully.

Don't listen to the anonymous cranks on the Internet. Ignore the Tweets and Facebook posts.

Don't listen to the friend or relative who says that you're just lazy, and not really struggling with an illness.

Trust yourself and the people closest to you with the truly important things in life: your mind, your heart, and your attention.

DO LISTEN TO TRUSTED FRIENDS

Speaking of the people closest to you, let's talk about friends, and why we should listen to them. Had I really listened to my dear friend Janell, for example, I might have saved myself years of misdiagnosis.

Janell had been through it all before me. When her father died in the '90s, Janell started gaining weight, her hair began falling out, and her hair and skin became dry.

Typical Janell, she immediately started pulling out medical textbooks, reading everything she could find, and she decided that her thyroid was probably out of whack. Her doctor told her she was just sad about losing her father, and he wanted to give her antidepressants. But Janell didn't buy it. She went back and forth—but a few months later, she finally insisted on a thyroid test. The doctor called her later with the results, and apologized over and over on the phone, telling her, "You were right. Your thyroid is in complete failure!"

When I was working on *Sheena,* Janell would come to Florida to visit me. At that time, Janell had also been diagnosed with celiac disease, but somehow, it didn't sink in. I kept thinking, what is all the talk about the thyroid? You hear *thyroid* being thrown around, and I never thought in a million years it was something I was struggling with. "Gena would have all these symptoms, mild depression, bloating, puffiness, weight gain, hair skin, and I said, 'I think you have something wrong with your thyroid. Seriously, you have the same symptoms I had.' But it's often hardest for people to listen to friends, and instead they put all their trust in a doctor."

If a friend who knows you and cares about you has advice, open your mind and listen. I wish I had. (And thanks, Janell, for not saying "I told you so!")

DON'T MISS OUT ON YOUR LIFE

John Lennon said, "Life is what happens to you while you're busy making other plans."

And if there's one thing I know, it's that even when you're struggling with a chronic disease, you want to do your best to live your life. But sometimes it's hard.

When I was a new mother, working on *Baywatch*, I was so tired and overworked that I never had enough time with Spencer. It was one of the reasons that I had to walk away from *Baywatch*. And I've never regretted that decision, because with Hudson and Stella, I've been able to be a stay-at-home mom. Yes, that's exhausting and tiring, too, but I don't feel that I've missed as much as I did with Spence.

My sister, Sheila, has commented on it, too. "I know Gena feels she missed out on a lot when Spencer was young. She was doing a lot of filming and traveling, reading lines, and trying to stay fit. With Hudson and Stella, she's been able to spend a lot of time with them, and is 100 percent hands-on."

I've sat at parks shaking, feeling sick and spacey, with dark circles under my eyes. I don't know how I was even able to drive sometimes. But I don't regret at least trying to do as much as I can for and with my children. I'm also lucky to have such a supportive husband who is such a great father to our children.

My struggle with thyroid disease has had an impact on my relationship with Cale at times as well. One year on our anniversary, we went away to a hotel without the children. It was so lovely to get away, to be able to sleep in. But I was sick the entire time. I was a bump on a log. Cale wanted to go to the pool and go to dinner, and I was just wishing we could rent a movie so I could stay in bed and rest. It's times like that when I feel like Debbie Downer.

So, try to do your best to participate, as much as you can. There may be days when you just can't muster enough energy, but always try.

But you also have to cut yourself some slack and forgive yourself, because as long as you try, people who love you do understand. Here's my son Spencer, talking about the times that I wasn't able to make it to games or events: "Before we found out about my mom's thyroid disease, I never took it personally if she couldn't make it to something, because I could see how tired she was. And after I found out my mom had the thyroid disease, I really felt bad for her. But she has always made an effort to be there for almost everything, and I really appreciate that about her."

DON'T LET OTHER PEOPLE DEFINE YOU

Whether I'm meeting someone at the kids' schools, or someone for a work project, or a doctor, I can usually tell right off the bat if they have some sort of preconceived ideas about me. Many people—not everyone—have some idea about my past, and unfortunately, with my having been on a show like *Baywatch*, and in *Playboy*, they jump to some pretty wild conclusions.

They figure I must be a bimbo . . . not particularly smart . . . a ditzy blonde. Maybe I was a wild party girl dating rocker dudes? Maybe I think I'm better than everyone else? Or perhaps I'm a spoiled princess who has had everything handed to her on a silver platter? Maybe I really *am* Neely Capshaw, and I'm plotting and planning how to steal husbands or blackmail them!

I'm none of these things, so I go into action, and make sure that other people don't get to define me, by making sure that my real self shines.

I do it by being myself.

When people meet me in person, they discover that I'm not usually what they expected. I have a goofy sense of humor—some of my friends even call me Lucy—after Lucille Ball. (And my brother calls me Oprah because he thinks I like to talk!)

I like to sew pillows and costumes for the kids, try new recipes, play on the beach with my family, watch Spencer play hockey, snuggle on the couch with Hank the dog, and go to dinner with my husband.

Sometimes at events, these Mr. Macho fans come up, usually carrying a copy of my *Playboy* spread for me to sign, and they start out with, "Hey, baby, whazzup" along with a lecherous look. Okay, I get it. They want to relate to me as a sex symbol. Not gonna happen! I throw them questions, ask them about a wife if I see a wedding ring. I ask them if they have kids. I get real, and quickly, because I only have a few seconds to do it. I'm able to quickly define my boundaries and redefine how they view me. And most of these guys, to be honest, end up posing for a photo with me, all smiles, and treating me like a sister or daughter or friend. You can see the respect. It's so gratifying!

Janell has always known this about me. "Gena is not a typical 'sex symbol.' She's a goofball, very silly and funny. Most of the time, what you notice is that she's happy, bubbly, making jokes. After they meet her in person, guys find her attractive because she's very natural, wholesome, and has that 'girl next door' vibe, more than anything. People love her not because she's beautiful, but because she has a big heart, she's smart as a whip, and funny as hell."

How do people try to define *you*? Are you part of the Mommy Wars—and if you're a stay-at-home mother, do mothers who work outside the home try to look down on you? Or, vice versa, if you're attractive, do people assume you're not smart? If you have a high-powered job, do people assume that you're not caring or nurturing? Do people try to pigeonhole you in ways that don't fit with the real you?

Figure out creative ways to help people quickly get the real you, set those boundaries, and get the respect you deserve!

LAUGH

One of life's automatic energy boosts is laughter. And I have to say, my friends always make me laugh. We've had so many adventures together that I could write a book just about those. Janell swears that I have good comedic timing.

We were at a convention in New Orleans, and one of *Sheena*'s producers took us to a wonderful nine-course dinner cooked by Emeril Lagasse himself. We went out clubbing that night and ran into actor Ray Romano, who we could see was getting a great deal of attention from female fans. The next day we were walking across the convention hall and we saw Ray.

"Hey, Ray," Gena shouted. "It's true what they say! Everybody *does* love Raymond!"

I do get off a good one sometimes!

I met my friend Jen in Scottsdale, at our sons' hockey games; we were the proverbial hockey moms. I remember we were sitting in the bleachers one day, and she was all excited. She had news to share!

"You know what?" She said. "I heard that there's a mom on this team who was on *Baywatch*!"

"Really, seriously?" I said.

"Yeah!" said Jen. "But I haven't seen her yet!"

"You're looking at her! It's me!" I said. We both collapsed in laughter.

They say laughter is the best medicine, and I have to agree!

SUNSET ON THE BEACH

I had a short time in the intense spotlight, but in the end, I know that it's hard to be real in the entertainment world. You're forever questioning who your friends are, whom you can trust. You never know if someone likes you, or wants to hang out with you because you're on the cover of a magazine or a TV show, or because they actually like you for you.

These days, I have a close circle of friends and family . . . people I can trust, people who love me for who I am. And I love them for who they are.

I'm embracing who I am and where I am. Now that I'm in my forties, I'm also letting go of all the expectations. The idea that I have to look a certain way, or weigh a certain amount, or be everything to everyone. Now I want to feel great and live a healthy life.

And the best part is that these days I feel sexier and more

beautiful as a woman than I did when I was twenty-five. Even in a swimsuit! I'm more focused on the inner life, the wisdom I've gained, what I've learned, my friends, my family, motherhood, and now, advocacy. I'm so much more of a woman now, compared to when I was running up and down that beach in my twenties. And, as one of my idols, Martha Stewart, would say, "That's a good thing."

Acknowledgments

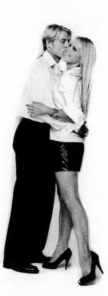

It is an obligation to tell one's story when it can potentially help others change their lives. That has been my outlook on this project from the beginning, to help others deal with what I've already been dealt. It's been a long journey, and I couldn't have done it without God's divine light and love, my family, friends, and the wonderful doctors and experts who all contributed to this book.

I first want to thank Cale, my husband, best friend, and co-parent, for his patience and encouragement during the writing of this book. We have such a special partnership that encompasses unconditional love and respect for one another, for that I am so grateful. Having a partner who's present and hands-on has given me the strength to push forward, find answers, and never give up. We've gone on to raise our children in a loving, honorable way that I'm so proud of. You embraced my illness with comfort and realistic expectations by picking up the slack when I simply couldn't. Whatever the challenge, you've always been right beside me in good times and in bad. You're the rock of our household and I thank God daily for the gift of our family and for the gift of you.

I thank my three beautiful children, Spencer, Hudson, and Stella, for supporting their mom and for being such great sports about sharing me with work, with writing this book, and with my advocacy. You kids are what make it all worthwhile as I watch each of you become the unique individuals you were meant to be. You make me so proud to be your mother every day of my life.

I thank my mother, Patricia, who did the best she could with what she had. God bless our parents, who walked through the trenches and came out with humble, loving hearts. That's my mom! We've been lucky enough to create a bond I didn't think possible. You've showed me what it takes to make things happen, to see the real meaning of life and the simplicity of it all. I have such deep respect for you as a woman, daughter, and mother. As you've always said, just BE, and everything will fall into place. I am doing just that, Mom.

I also want to thank my sister, Sheila, and brother, Michael, for their love and support. Regardless of the geographic distance between us, you've always made a point to stay close and be present in our lives. The relationship you have with my children is beyond words and fills my heart with such joy. I thank you both for that. Sheila, sorry for wearing your clothes without asking as a tween, and Michael, well . . . just sorry! (We had some really good scraps as kids.) I love you guys so much!

I want to especially thank Mary Shomon for helping to create the opportunity for me to make a difference in writing this book. I have such profound respect for you both personally and professionally. Mary, you are a true inspiration and an example to us all by the way you give of your time and in the books you write. You've helped so many find their way, including myself. Thank you for this gift of collaboration and for your dear friendship. Also, special thanks to Gail Dana and Dan Shomon for being such exceptional hosts while we were in Tampa for our first writing session. Our morning conversations over coffee and fresh fruit made me feel right at home.

I thank my administrator and friend Linda Adams for her partnership on the Thyroid Sexy Facebook page. I couldn't do it without you. Your unbelievable wealth of knowledge and soulful heart shines on the pages and warms the hearts of us all. We get each other's humor and have such a blast running TS! Your song, "Thyroid Blues," is testament to your musical talent and passion for thyroid advocacy. Thank you, Thysista!

Thank you, Dr. Alan Christianson, for your incredible thyroid knowledge and giving heart. I've enjoyed our Thyroid Sexy boot camps and creating thyroid awareness together. You have a beautiful energy that puts your patients at ease, and you listen and treat the symptoms! We always seem to get "on track" and it's simply because you're a wonderful doctor. It must be our Minnesota roots and all that wild rice, because we click!

Thanks to my amazing attorney, Mark Kalmonshon. Twenty years and counting, what a ride it's been, and a great one at that. Thank you for always having my back and getting things done!

I thank our agent, Carol Mann, for making this dream of mine a reality! It all started with a little Facebook page. Now I'm telling my Thyroid Sexy story center stage, Broadway-style, and I thank you dearly.

I thank our editor, Sarah Durand, at Simon & Schuster. You understood what this book meant to us and that the word *sexy* can be related to our thyroids. We're creating awareness in a way that's never been done before, thanks to you.

Thank you to the incredible Sara Gottfried, MD, who contributed the Foreword, and so many wonderful ideas for the book. Sara, you're changing the world for women!

Thanks also to all the doctors and experts who contributed to our book: Alan Christianson, ND; David Borenstein, MD; Kent Holtorf, MD; Richard Shames, MD; Karilee Shames, RN, PhD; and Kevin Passero, ND.

Thanks also to Teresa Tapp, Lisa Moretti, and Lauren Lucernoni for your help and support.

Special thanks to the following family, friends, and contributors for their support:

Cale Hulse, Spencer Fahlman, Caia Hulse, Hudson Hulse, Stella Hulse, Patricia Nolin, Sheila Sutton, Michael Olsen, Grandma Marie Rodgers, David and Lorraine Hulse, Janell Martin, Becky Newell, Jennifer Winslow, Greg Fahlman, Keith Ricks, Jerry Shandrew, Barbara Teszler PR, Keith and Chantal Tkachuk, Phyliss Lane, Gary Quinn, Ken Baker, Kristi Kaylor, Torrie Wilson, Nancy Archeletta, Doug and Debbie Schwartz, Michael Berk, Bob Barker, David Hasselhoff, Greg Bonann, Tara Hitchcock, Nancy and Nels Van Patten, Rachel Hunter, Rona Menashe, Alicia Arden, Kim Alaspa, Zev Forrest, Stephen Baldwin, Anne Lange, *AND* to all the "Sexies" who inspire me everyday! Thank you!

I would like to especially thank Christie Brinkley and Alec Baldwin for their support and friendship, and support of my Thyroid Sexy page and community.

—Gena Lee Nolin

I must thank my family, including my wonderful children, Julia and Danny. You both were so patient and supportive as I worked on this book. You are my joy and my heart, and you always keep things interesting! Thanks to my father, Dan Shomon, and brother, Dan Shomon Jr.—you both are always there for me. Many thanks also to my father's fiancée, Gail Dana. Gail, you and Dad opened your home to Gena and me for our intensive writing session, and your loving care and comfy home made for a relaxing and productive place for us to work. I love you all!

As always I am so grateful for my agent, Carol Mann, who believed in this book and provided such excellent guidance and moral support all the way through. I'm also thrilled to be back with my first editor, the top-notch Sarah Durand. Sarah, you always make a book better in so many ways, and it's a pleasure to work with you, and the terrific Daniella Wexler. Thanks also to PR guru Barbara Teszler for your sharp advice and support.

Thank you to the superb practitioners who have shared their knowledge, expertise, and support, starting first of all with my dear friend and colleague Sara Gottfried, MD, who is a role model in every way for today's savvy, successful, healthy women.

I also want to thank Alan Christianson, ND; David Borenstein, MD; Kent Holtorf, MD; Richard Shames, MD; Karilee Shames, RN, PhD; and Kevin Passero, ND. All thyroid patients should be so lucky as to have any of you to guide them on the path to wellness.

Thanks to thyroid advocates Linda Adams, Geri Rybacki, Katie Schwartz, Dana Trentini, and Robert Chapman, for your tireless efforts on behalf of the thyroid community and your unflagging support for this book.

A special thank-you to Jane Frank. Jane, you are not only the best friend a girl could have, but you have been such a tremendous help in my business. And thanks, too, to Lauren Lucernoni and Rita Roman for your research help.

Two very special friends are always there with love, support, and their special brand of magic—Teresa Tapp and Lisa Moretti. T and Lisa—you are the best!

And where would I be without some dear, dear friends who are smart, caring, supportive, and insightful? So, thank you, Julia Schopick, Rebecca Elia, Genevieve Piturro, Demo DiMartile, Mohammed Antabli, Franca Fiabane, Kim Conley, Laura Horton, Debbie Mulhern, Darcy Shoop, and Julia Szabo.

Gena is blessed to have a wonderful family and amazing friends. It was a pleasure to get to know them over the course of writing this book. Special thanks go out to Cale Hulse, Patricia Nolin, Sheila Sutton, Janell Martin, Becky Newell, Greg Fahlman, and Spencer Fahlman. You are all lucky to have Gena in your life, and Gena is lucky to have you.

And of course, I want to thank the incredible Gena Lee Nolin. Gena, you are courageous, hilarious, and one of the most compassionate people I've ever met. You have fearlessly shared your story, and you are willing to stick your neck out—pun intended!—for your fellow thyroid patients. You are truly a beautiful person, inside and out, and I am fortunate to count you among my friends.

—Mary Shomon

Resources

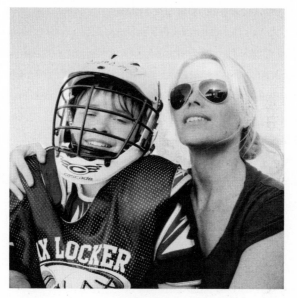

With Spencer

BEAUTIFUL INSIDE AND OUT
ON THE WEB

http://www.beautifulinsideandoutbook.com
Home page for the book, including resources, links, checklists, and more.

Also, http://www.facebook.com/beautifulinsideandoutbook

THYROID SEXY COMMUNITY

Thyroid Sexy

http://www.thyroidsexy.com

Home page for the community and thyroid advocacy campaign.

Thyroid Sexy on Facebook

http://www.facebook.com/thyroidsexy

The Facebook community of Thyroid Sexy readers and supporters, where Gena Lee Nolin interacts and shares her thyroid journeys, support, and experiences with other thyroid patients, and patients support each other with advice and compassion.

Thyroid Sexy on Twitter

http://www.twitter.com/thyroidsexy

The Twitter feed for the Thyroid Sexy book and advocacy campaign.

GENA LEE NOLIN ONLINE

The Official Gena Lee Nolin Site

http://www.officialgenaleenolin.com

Gena Lee Nolin's official website, featuring her filmography, photos, blog, and latest news.

Gena Lee Nolin on WhoSay

http://www.whosay.com/genaleenolin

Gena Lee Nolin's page/blog on the popular celebrity site WhoSay.

Gena Lee Nolin on Facebook
https://www.facebook.com/pages/Gena-Lee-Nolin
 /171537890368
Gena Lee Nolin's Facebook page, where she interacts with fans and shares her latest news.

Gena Lee Nolin on Twitter
http://www.twitter.com/genaleenolin
Gena's personal Twitter feed, where she shares her thoughts, observations, and latest news.

MARY SHOMON'S SITES, RESOURCES, BOOKS

Thyroid-Info.com
http://www.thyroid-info.com
The home page for Mary Shomon's patient advocacy efforts, books, articles, and newsletters.

Mary Shomon's Thyroid Support on Facebook
http://www.facebook.com/thyroidsupport
An active thyroid support community, where Mary shares articles, links, and information, and thyroid patients support each other.

About.com Thyroid Site
http://thyroid.about.com
The site that Mary has guided since 1996 that is one of the Internet's hottest spots for the latest thyroid news, articles, information, and advocacy.

Mary Shomon on Twitter

http://www.twitter.com/thyroidmary

Thyroid Diet

http://www.facebook.com/thyroiddiet
An online community for thyroid patients focused on metabolism, healthy diet, and weight loss.

Thyroid Diet Revolution

http://www.thyroiddietrevolution.com
This site features Mary Shomon's *New York Times* bestselling book *The Thyroid Diet Revolution: Manage Your Master Gland of Metabolism for Lasting Weight Loss.*

Thyroid Coaching Sessions with Mary Shomon

http://www.thyroidcoaching.com
Email: coaching@thyroid-info.com
Phone: 888-810-9471; 301-493-6109
Home page for Mary Shomon's personal telephone coaching services with thyroid and hormone patients.

Other Books by Mary Shomon

Living Well with Hypothyroidism: What Your Doctor Doesn't Tell You . . . That You Need to Know, 2nd Edition. New York: HarperCollins.
http://www.thyroid-info.com/book.htm

Living Well with Graves' Disease and Hyperthyroidism: What Your Doctor Doesn't Tell You . . . That You Need to Know. New York: HarperCollins.
http://www.thyroid-info.com/graves

The Menopause Thyroid Solution: Overcoming Menopause by Solving Your Hidden Thyroid Problems. New York: HarperCollins.
http://www.menopausethyroid.com

The Thyroid Hormone Breakthrough: Overcoming Sexual and Hormonal Problems at Every Age. New York: HarperCollins.
http://www.thyroidbreakthrough.com

Thyroid Guide to Hair Loss: Conventional and Holistic Help for People Suffering Thyroid-Related Hair Loss. Seattle: CreateSpace Independent Publisher Platform.
http://www.thyroid-info.com/hair

Living Well With Autoimmune Disease: What Your Doctor Doesn't Tell You . . . That You Need to Know. New York: HarperCollins

Living Well with Chronic Fatigue Syndrome and Fibromyalgia: What Your Doctor Doesn't Tell You . . . That You Need to Know. New York: HarperCollins.

THYROID AND ENDOCRINOLOGY ORGANIZATIONS

National Academy of Hypothyroidism
http://www.nahypothyroidism.org
Founded by Kent Holtorf, MD, this group seeks to improve the quality of diagnosis and treatment of hypothyroidism through research and education with both the medical and patient communities.

Coalition for Better Thyroid Care

http://www.betterthyroidcare.org

http://www.facebook.com/BetterThyroidCare

The Coalition for Better Thyroid Care, a patient-driven organization created in 2010, promotes improvements in thyroid care and provides information on thyroid tests and treatment options.

American Autoimmune Related Diseases Association

http://www.aarda.org

Phone: 810-776-3900

22100 Gratiot Avenue, East Detroit, MI 48021

AARDA provides information about more than fifty different autoimmune disorders, including Hashimoto's disease and Graves' disease. This website and organization provide general information about autoimmune disorders and profiles of specific diseases.

American Association of Clinical Endocrinologists

http://www.aace.com

Phone: 904-353-7878; Fax: 904-353-8185

1000 Riverside Avenue, Suite 205, Jacksonville, FL 32204

The American Association of Clinical Endocrinologists (AACE) is a professional medical organization devoted to clinical endocrinology. They sponsor an online Specialist Search Page at http://www.aace.com/directory, which allows you to identify AACE members by geographic location, including international options. A unique feature of this page is the ability to select by subspecialty.

American Thyroid Association

http://www.thyroid.org

Patient Information Line: 800-THYROID (800-849-7643)

Phone: 703-998-8890; Fax: 703-998-8893

6066 Leesburg Pike, PO Box 1836, Falls Church, VA 22041

Founded in 1923, ATA promotes scientific and public understanding of the biology of the thyroid gland and its disorders, so as to improve methods for prevention, diagnosis, and management of thyroid disease.

Thyroid Foundation of Canada/La Fondation Canadienne de la Thyroide

http://www.thyroid.ca

Phone: (Canada) 519-649-5478, 800-267-8822; Fax: 519-649-5402

1669 Jalna Blvd., Suite 803, London, Ontario N6E 3S1

Established in 1980, Thyroid Foundation of Canada was the first thyroid patient organization in the world. The volunteer-run foundation offers information for thyroid patients and interested practitioners, in English and French.

The Endocrine Society

http://www.endo-society.org

Email: endostaff@endo-society.org

Phone: 301-941-0200; Fax: 301-941-0259

8401 Connecticut Avenue, Suite 900, Chevy Chase, MD 20815-5817

A group with a mission promoting the understanding of hormones and endocrinology, and the impact of this knowledge on preventing, diagnosing, and treating disease, including thyroid disease and obesity. The group publishes a number of journals and maintains an informational website.

Hormone Foundation

http://www.hormone.org

Phone: 800-HORMONE (800-467-6663)

8401 Connecticut Avenue, Suite 900, Chevy Chase, MD 20815-5817

The Hormone Foundation, the public education affiliate of The Endocrine Society, is a leading source of hormone-related health information for the public, physicians, allied health professionals, and the media.

Thyroid UK

http://www.thyroiduk.org

Phone: 01255 820407

32, Darcy Road, St Osyth, Clacton on Sea, Essex, UK CO16 8QF

Lyn Mynott is the chair and chief executive of this patient-oriented organization helping raise awareness of thyroid issues, and improve the level of thyroid care in the United Kingdom.

OTHER RECOMMENDED THYROID SITES

Elaine Moore's Graves' Disease Site

http://www.elaine-moore.com

Thyroid Disease Manager

http://www.thyroidmanager.org

DearThyroid

http://www.dearthyroid.org

Richard Shames, MD, and Karilee Shames, PhD, RN

http://www.thyroidmindpower.com

Jacob Teitelbaum, MD
http://www.endfatigue.com

Holtorf Medical Group
http://www.holtorfmed.com

SOCIAL MEDIA AND BLOGS

Who to Follow on Twitter for Thyroid Info

A few key folks to follow if you want to stay up on thyroid issues on Twitter:

- Endocrine Today / @EndocrineToday—This Twitter account sends out updates that help you stay up on Endocrine Today's useful website, which features the latest endocrine and thyroid news.
- EndocrineWeb / @endocrineweb—EndocrineWeb sends out useful information related to thyroid and hormonal health.
- Kent Holtorf, MD / @HoltorfMed—Kent Holtorf, MD, is an integrative physician with specialization in thyroid and hormone balance, and founder of the Holtorf Medical Center network of practices around the country.
- Sara Gottfried, MD / @DrGottfried—Sara Gottfried, MD is a Harvard-trained holistic gynecologist, yogi, and mom who focuses on thyroid and hormone health and balance, healthy nutrition, and holistic lifestyle issues.
- Thyroid Cancer Survivor's Association (ThyCa) / @ ThyCaInc—The official Thyroid Cancer Survivor's

Association Twitter account stays up on thyroid cancer and related news and support information.

- Friends of the American Thyroid Association / @ThyroidFriends—A group that provides support information from the American Thyroid Association (ATA).
- Dear Thyroid / @DearThyroid—The Dear Thyroid community for thyroid support is active on Twitter, sharing information, humor, support, and links. (Read an interview with founder Katie Schwartz.)
- Robert the HypoMan / @Hypo_Man-Robert is a sharp, UK-based thyroid patient with heart, who provides valuable links to content, as well as interactive support on Twitter. (Read more at www.hypoman.com.)
- Hypothyroid Mom / @HypothyroidMom—A Mom with hypothyroidism, looking at being healthy, being a good mother, sharing links and being an advocate with a unique perspective.

Following Us on Twitter

Gena Lee Nolin / @ThyroidSexy

Mary Shomon / @ThyroidMary

Some of Our Favorite Thyroid Blogs

Mary Shomon's Blog—http://www.thyroid-info.com

Dana Trentini / Hypothyroid Mom—http://www
.hypothyroidmom.com

Elaine Moore—http://www.elaine-moore.com/

Robert Chapman, aka HypoMan—http://www.hypoman.com

Carol Gray, aka Crazy Thyroid Lady—http://
crazythyroidlady.blogspot.com/

DearThyroid—http://www.dearthyroid.com

About.com Thyroid Blog—http://thyroid.about.com/b

TESTING LABORATORIES

MyMedLab

http://www.thyroid-info.com/mymedlab

Phone: 888-MYMEDLAB (888-696-3352)

Through MyMedLab, patients can order almost any thyroid or hormone blood test or panel, without a doctor's prescription, at wholesale costs with minimal markup. Have your blood drawn at one of thousands of LabCorp locations and other collection laboratories around the country, and get the results sent directly to you by mail and online.

ZRT Laboratory

http://www.salivatest.com

Phone: 503-466-2445; Fax: 503 466-1636; Hormone Hotline: 503-466-9166

1815 NW 169th Place Suite 5050, Beaverton, OR 97006

Diagnos-Techs, Inc.

http://www.diagnostechs.com

Phone: 800-878-3787

Clinical and Research Laboratory, 6620 S. 192nd Place, Bldg. J, Kent, WA 98032

Genova Diagnostics (Formerly Great Smokies Diagnostic Laboratory)

http://www.genovadiagnostics.com

Phone: 800-522-4762, 828-253-0621

63 Zillicoa Street, Asheville, NC 28801

Saliva hormone testing for estradiol, estrone, estriol, progesterone, and testosterone, in a variety of panels. Available only
through your health care provider.

THYROID DRUGS AND THEIR MANUFACTURERS

Levoxyl, Cytomel, Tapazole

Levoxyl is a levothyroxine product. Cytomel is liothyronine, the
synthetic form of triiodothyronine (T3). Tapazole is the brand
name for the antithyroid drug methimazole.

King Pharmaceuticals, Inc.

http://www.kingpharm.com

Phone: 800-776-3637; 423-989-8000

501 Fifth Street, Bristol, TN 37620

Levoxyl

http://www.levoxyl.com

Phone: 866-LEVOXYL (866-538-6995)

Cytomel

http:// www.kingpharm.com

Tapazole

http:// www.kingpharm.com

Armour Thyroid, Thyrolar, Levothroid
Armour Thyroid is a natural thyroid hormone replacement product. Levothroid is a levothyroxine drug.

Forest Pharmaceuticals
http://www.forestpharm.com
Phone: 800-678-1605, ext.7301; Fax: 314-493-7457
Professional Affairs Department, 13600 Shoreline Drive, St. Louis, MO 63045

Armour Thyroid
http://www.armourthyroid.com

Levothroid
http://www.levothroid.com

Unithroid
Phone: 800-325-9994, 215-333-9000
A brand of levothyroxine distributed by Lannett Pharmaceuticals, 9000 State Road, Philadelphia, PA 19136

Nature-Throid/Westhroid
Nature-Throid and Westhroid are prescription desiccated thyroid drugs. Westhroid is a cornstarch-bound, natural thyroid hormone product. Nature-Throid is bound with microcrystalline cellulose, and is hypoallergenic.

RLC Laboratories
http://www.rlclabs.com/
Phone: 877-797-7997
28248 North Tatum Blvd, Suite B1-629, Cave Creek, AZ 85331

Nature-Throid
http://www.nature-throid.com

Westhroid
http://www.westhroidp.com

Synthroid
http://www.synthroid.com
http://abbott.com
Phone: 800-255-5162
Abbott Laboratories, 100 Abbott Park Road, Abbott Park, IL
  60064-3500
Synthroid is the top-selling levothyroxine drug.

Tirosint
Tirosint is a gel capsule form of levothyroxine.

Akrimax Pharmaceuticals, LLC
http://www.tirosintgelcaps.com
Phone: 1-908-372-0506
11 Commerce Drive, 1st Floor, Suite 100, Cranford, NJ 07016

Thyrogen
http://www.thyrogen.com
Phone: 800-745-4447; 617-768-9000
Genzyme Therapeutics, 500 Kendall Street, Cambridge, MA
  02142
Thyrogen is a drug that, when used along with tests to detect recurrent or leftover thyroid cancer, can prevent the need to become
hypothyroid as part of that testing.

HERBS/SUPPLEMENT INFORMATION

iHerb

http://www.iherb.com

An excellent website for a variety of diet foods, low-carb products, vitamins, and supplements at low cost.

Consumer Lab

http://www.consumerlab.com

This site is a great resource for people interested in taking herbal supplements. ConsumerLab.com offers independent testing of popular herbs to help consumers evaluate the safety of vitamins, minerals, herbal products, and more.

EXERCISE/MOVEMENT

T-Tapp

http://www.t-tapp.com

Phone: 800-342-0717

Teresa Tapp's exercise program has taken the United States and Canada by storm. Innovative and successful, the exercises rely upon a creative approach to bending, stretching, isometrics, and careful standing and walking postures that can be done by anyone, at any age, weight, or level of fitness. The programs are available on DVDs and are designed to be done anywhere: home, office, or workplace.

BEAUTY/BEAUTY PRODUCT WEBSITES

***Beauty Addict* Blog**

http://beautyaddict.blogspot.com/

This beauty blog is updated with the latest happenings in the world of skin, body, and hair care. It also features a wide range of topics from celebrities and fashion to beauty treatments.

Sephora
http://www.sephora.com/
If you're looking for a wide range of beauty products, you'll enjoy Sephora. From hard-to-find brands to the latest trends, Sephora's website has more than 12,000 beauty products and counting.

Beauty at iVillage
http://www.ivillage.com/beauty-style
This glossy and stylish site offers celebrity gossip and beauty tips.

***Elle* Magazine**
http://www.elle.com/beauty/
Elle magazine online features fashion, style, and popular reviews of beauty products.

GLUTEN-FREE RESOURCES

Informational Websites
Celiac
http://www.celiac.com
Celiac.com was founded in 1995 by Scott Adams, coauthor of the book *Cereal Killers*, founder and publisher of *Journal of Gluten Sensitivity*, and founder and owner of The Gluten Free Mall. Adams has a single goal for the site: to help as many people as possible with celiac disease get diagnosed and living a happy, healthy, gluten-free life.

G-Free Foodie
http://www.gfreefoodie.com/
G-Free Foodie is a website for people who love food and live gluten free. This website contains recipes, product conversions, kid menu options, product reviews, articles, blogs, and restaurants. This website has a great restaurant locator resource. Click on the restaurant tab and type in your zip code to find pages of gluten-free restaurants in your area.

Gluten-Free Girl Blog
http://www.glutenfreegirl.com/
The author of this site has celiac disease and offers many tips on preparing and eating tasty gluten-free food. Her blog is a mix of recipes, her own experiences, and videos on how to create great gluten-free recipes.

Where to Purchase Gluten-Free Foods
Your Local Supermarket or Health Food Store
Ask the managers of your local supermarket to carry special products for you to purchase at your convenience. Health food stores are also a great source for gluten-free or specialty health products. Around the country, the chains Publix, Shoprite, Stop & Shop, Giant, Trader Joe's, and Whole Food, among others, have good selections of gluten-free products.

Amazon
http://www.amazon.com/grocery
The Amazon website offers the ability to purchase a wide variety of gluten-free foods and ship them to your own home.

Gluten Free Mall

http://www.celiac.com/glutenfreemall/

The Celiac.com site maintains the Gluten Free Mall, an online source for a variety of gluten-free products.

GlutenFree.com

http://www.glutenfree.com

Glutenfree.com carries a broad range of gluten-free products, including popular brands like Glutino, Bakery on Main, Mary's Gone Crackers, and more.

Other Gluten-Free Favorites

Chex Gluten Free Cereals

http://www.chex.com/GlutenFree

Udi's Bread

http://udisfood.com

Rudi's Bakery

http://www.rudisbakery.com

Blue Diamond Nut Thins Crackers

http://www.bluediamond.com

Pamela's Gluten-Free Products

http://www.pamelasproducts.com

Mary's Gone Crackers Products

http://www.marysgonecrackers.com

OUR FAVORITE BEAUTY PRODUCTS

Hair and Hair Care

Hair Extensions by Jessica Simpson/Ken Paves
http://shopkenpaves.com
http://www.hairextensions.com/hairdo.html

Hairstylist Brent Hardgrave
http://brenthardgrave.com
Phone: 678-777-1099
Email: brent@brenthardgrave.com

Simplicity Hair Extensions / Tressallure
http://www.simplicityhair.com

Tabatha Coffey's Luxhair How Extensions
http://www.luxhair.com/brand/how

Kérastase Paris Hair Care
http://www.kerastase-usa.com

Aveeno
http://www.aveeno.com

Pantene
http://www.pantene.com

Lashes and Eyebrows
Rapidlash
https://www.rapidlash.com/

Anastasia Beverly Hills
http://www.anastasia.net/

Sephora Eyebrow Kit
http://www.sephora.com

Cosmetics
Chanel Cosmetics
http://www.chanel.com/

Urban Decay Cosmetics
http://www.urbandecay.com/

NARS Cosmetics
http://www.narscosmetics.com

MAC Cosmetics
http://www.maccosmetics.com

Skin Care
Ole Henriksen Skin Care
http://www.olehenriksen.com/

Kiehl's Skin Care Products
http://www.kiehls.com

Peter Thomas Roth Clinical Skin Care Products
http://www.peterthomasroth.com

NeriumAD
http://www.maryshomon.nerium.com

Fragrances

Thierry Mugler

http://www.muglerstoreusa.com

Clive Christian

http://www.clive.com/

CELEBRITY NEWS

E! Online News

http://www.eonline.com/

Based in Los Angeles, E! Online was launched in 1996 as the comprehensive entertainment news website. Today, E! Online has more than 20,000 entertainment news stories archived on the site, making it an unparalleled resource for celebrity-driven entertainment information.

***People* Magazine**

http://www.people.com/people/

Website for the popular celebrity magazine, featuring celebrity news, behind-the-scenes candids, and loads of exclusives you won't find anywhere else.

Oh No They Didn't!

http://ohnotheydidnt.livejournal.com/

Oh No They Didn't! (ONTD for short) is a community-driven celebrity gossip site, with members submitting items from all sorts of entertainment venues (gaming, music, breaking news, celebrities, scandals, etc.) throughout the day.

PopSugar

http://www.popsugar.com

Celebrity news on favorite stars at PopSugar, a witty site that pokes gentle fun at Hollywood. There is breaking content here as well as thoughtful features.

HuffPost Entertainment

http://www.huffingtonpost.com/entertainment/

Features the latest celebrity news, blog posts from celebrities, and Hollywood coverage.

MOTHERHOOD AND FAMILY LIFE

Modern Mom

http://www.modernmom.com/

A comprehensive site, ModernMom.com features smart practical tips and advice on topics such as parenting, pregnancy, family, cooking, finances, career, health, wellness, beauty, entertainment, and more.

Motherhood Café

http://www.motherhood-cafe.com/

Created by a mom and PhD in sociology and specializing in parenting culture, Motherhood Café is a trusted community where mothers can get perspective, as well as helpful knowledge and information about their parenting experiences and concerns.

Plugged In Parents

http://www.pluggedinparents.com

A comprehensive cyberworld that offers advice from a pediatric nurse practitioner, reader-approved recipes, and even family-dog pros and cons.

Working Mother
http://www.workingmother.com/
Working Mother Media's mission is to serve as a champion of culture change. WorkingMother.com gives working mothers advice for home and work.

Babble
http://www.babble.com/
Babble says it's "for a new generation of parents," and it looks at various aspects of parenting with a contemporary eye.

FINDING DOCTORS AND PRACTITIONERS, VERIFYING CREDENTIALS

Mary Shomon's Thyroid Top Doctors Directory
http://www.thyroid-info.com/topdrs

American Association of Clinical Endocrinologists Database
http://www.aace.com/memsearch.php

American Thyroid Association's Find a Thyroid Specialist Database
http://www.thyroid.org/patients/specialists.php3

American Osteopathic Association
http://www.aoa-net.org
Phone: 800-621-1773; 312-202-8000; Fax 312-202-8200
142 East Ontario Street, Chicago, IL 60611

American Academy of Osteopathy

Find a Physician page-http://www.academyofosteopathy.org/ findphys.cfm

Phone: 317-879-1881

3500 DePauw Blvd., Suite 1080, Indianapolis, IN 46268

The Cranial Academy

Find a Professional-http://www.cranialacademy.com/ agreement.html

Phone: 317-594-0411, 317-594-9299

8202 Clearvista Parkway #9D, Indianapolis, IN 46256

American Board of Integrative Holistic Medicine

http://www.holisticboard.org/D/locate_physician.html

Phone: 509-886-3046

614 Daniel Drive NE, East Wenachee, WA, 98802-4036

American Holistic Health Association Referrals

http://ahha.org/referrals.asp

Phone: 714-779-6152

PO Box 17400, Anaheim, CA 92817-7400

American Holistic Medical Association Doctor Finder

http://www.holisticmedicine.org

Phone: 216-292-6644

27629 Chagrin Blvd., Suite 206, Woodmere, OH 44122

PRACTITIONERS FEATURED IN THE BOOK

David Borenstein, MD

http://www.davidborensteinmd.com

Phone: 212-262-2412

Manhattan Integrative Medicine, PC, 1841 Broadway (at 60th Street), Suite 1012, New York, NY 10023

Integrative physician with expertise in hormone balance, thyroid treatment, cancer support, and rehabilitative medicine.

Alan Christianson, ND

http://www.integrativehealthcare.com

info@integrativehealthcare.com

Phone: 480-657-0003

9200 East Raintree Drive, Suite 100, Scottsdale, AZ 85260

Naturopathic care of hormone, thyroid and immune imbalances, and weight loss.

Sara Gottfried, MD

http://www.GottfriedCenter.com

http://twitter.com/DrGottfried

http://drgottfried.blogspot.com

Phone: 510-893-3907

Gottfried Center for Integrative Medicine, 300 Lakeside Drive, Suite 202, Oakland, CA 94612

Integrative gynecologist, hormone expert, author, blogger, and founder and medical director of the Gottfried Center.

Kent Holtorf, MD

http://www.holtorfmed.com

Phone: 310-375-2705

Holtorf Medical Group, 23456 Hawthorne Blvd. Suite #160, Torrance, CA 90505

Hormone, thyroid, and weight loss expert; founder of the Holtorf Medical Group and the National Academy of Hypothyroidism.

Kevin Passero, ND

http://www.healthtides.com

Phone: 443-433-5540

Offices in Washington, DC; Annapolis, MD; and Bethesda, MD

Founder of Green Healing Wellness Center, specializing in hormone balance, thyroid treatment, and holistic mental health.

Richard Shames, MD, and Karilee Halo Shames, RN, PhD

http://www.thyroidmindpower.com

Phone: 415-472-2343; Fax: 415-472-7636

PO Box 2466, Sebastopol, CA 95473

Holistic, integrative health practice, telephone consulting, office practice, authors of *Thyroid Power: Ten Steps to Feeling Power; Feeling Fat, Fuzzy, or Frazzled? A Three-Step Program to: Restore Thyroid, Adrenal, And Reproductive Balance, Beat Hormone Havoc, and Feel Better Fast!; and Thyroid Mind Power: The Proven Cure for Hormone-Related Depression, Anxiety, and Memory Loss*

Index